A WHO Public Health Approach to Ending AIDs in the Global South

In highlighting how a WHO Public Health Approach (PHA) has been successfully used in developing countries to provide HIV/AIDS patients with antiretroviral therapy (ART), this important book provides a template for how the PHA can be implemented to treat other chronic but non-communicable diseases (NCDs) as well. With over 28 million people globally now receiving treatment for HIV/AIDS, it's clear there are lessons to be learnt from the provision of ART which have great relevance for NCD care and towards achieving universal health coverage in the global south.

The first section of the book provides a detailed overview of the strategy that enabled such a successful programme to be taken place, the challenges faced and its evolution over time. The book then moves on to assert that by approaching other chronic NCDs in a similar way, focussing on populations with integrated long-term and short-term person-centred care, there is a pathway towards universal healthcare and Universal Health Coverage across the developing world.

Discussing many of the most pressing diseases and public health issues affecting these regions, this book provides global health scholars and practitioners with a detailed analysis of the challenges faced in tackling these diseases, but also an integrated person-centred health-care approach by which these challenges may be met.

Charles F. Gilks holds the inaugural Queensland Professorial Chair in Blood-borne Viruses and STIs at the University of Queensland (UQ). He is a global health specialist and clinical academic. A UK graduate, he started working on HIV/AIDS in East Africa in 1988, based in Nairobi at the Kenya Medical Research Institute. He became the Professor of Tropical Medicine at the Liverpool School of Tropical Medicine in 1994 before moving to WHO in 2001 to head up HIV treatment and prevention scale-up and to drive "3by5" roll out. He was appointed UNAIDS Country Coordinator in India in 2009 and moved to Australia in 2013 to become Dean and Head of the School of Public Health at UQ.

Yibeltal Assefa Alemu is an Associate Professor in Global Health Systems at the School of Public Health, the University of Queensland. He has played key roles in developing national and global guidelines and contributed to health systems strengthening and universal health coverage in Ethiopia and other resource-limited settings. He has held influential positions in Ethiopia, including Deputy Director General of the Ethiopian Public Health Institute, Executive Director of the International Institute for Primary Health Care, Director of Medical Services at the Federal Ministry of Health, Director of Planning, Monitoring and Evaluation as well as Head of Health Programs at the Federal HIV/AIDS Prevention and Control Office.

A WHO Public Health Approach to Ending AIDS in the Global South

Lessons for NCD Control and Universal Health Coverage

Charles F. Gilks and Yibeltal Assefa Alemu

Routledge
Taylor & Francis Group
LONDON AND NEW YORK

First published 2025
by Routledge
4 Park Square, Milton Park, Abingdon, Oxon OX14 4RN

and by Routledge
605 Third Avenue, New York, NY 10158

Routledge is an imprint of the Taylor & Francis Group, an informa business

British Library Cataloguing-in-Publication Data
A catalogue record for this book is available from the British Library

Library of Congress Cataloging-in-Publication Data
Names: Gilks, Charles F., author. | Alemu, Yibeltal, author.
Title: A WHO public health approach to ending AIDS in the global south / Charles Gilks and Yibeltal Alemu.
Description: Abingdon, Oxon ; New York, NY : Routledge, 2024. | Includes bibliographical references and index.
Identifiers: LCCN 2024011170 (print) | LCCN 2024011171 (ebook) | ISBN 9781032342337 (hardback) | ISBN 9781032826905 (paperback) | ISBN 9781003505693 (ebook)
Subjects: MESH: World Health Organization. | Public Health Practice | HIV Infections—prevention & control | Acquired Immunodeficiency Syndrome—prevention & control | Noncommunicable Diseases | Universal Health Insurance | Developing Countries | Social Determinants of Health Classification: LCC RC606.6 .G54 2024 (print) | LCC RC606.6 (ebook) | NLM WA 100 | DDC 362.19697/92—dc23/eng/20240329
LC record available at https://lccn.loc.gov/2024011170
LC ebook record available at https://lccn.loc.gov/2024011171

ISBN: 978-1-032-34233-7 (hbk)
ISBN: 978-1-032-82690-5 (pbk)
ISBN: 978-1-003-50569-3 (ebk)

DOI: 10.4324/9781003505693

Typeset in Times New Roman
by codeMantra

To Marina and Birtukan (Blen), for all their love and inspiration. Our book would have been impossible without their support.

Contents

Author biographies

Charles F. Gilks holds the inaugural Queensland Professorial Chair in Blood-borne Viruses and STIs at the University of Queensland (UQ). He is a global health specialist and clinical academic. A UK graduate, he started working on HIV/AIDS in East Africa in 1988, based in Nairobi at the Kenya Medical Research Institute. He became the Professor of Tropical Medicine at the Liverpool School of Tropical Medicine in 1994 before moving to WHO in 2001 to head up HIV treatment and prevention scale-up and to drive "3by5" roll out. He was appointed UNAIDS Country Coordinator in India in 2009 and moved to Australia in 2013 to become Dean and Head of the School of Public Health at UQ.

Yibeltal Assefa Alemu is an Associate Professor in Global Health Systems at the School of Public Health, the University of Queensland. He has played key roles in developing national and global guidelines and contributed to health systems strengthening and universal health coverage in Ethiopia and other resource-limited settings. He has held influential positions in Ethiopia, including Deputy Director General of the Ethiopian Public Health Institute, Executive Director of the International Institute for Primary Health Care, Director of Medical Services at the Federal Ministry of Health, Director of Planning, Monitoring and Evaluation as well as Head of Health Programs at the Federal HIV/AIDS Prevention and Control Office.

Foreword

The world has made remarkable progress in the response to HIV and AIDS. Much of this success can be attributed to the public health approach adopted across the world to secure access to life-saving antiretroviral therapy (ART) which has revolutionised HIV prevention, treatment and care.

The key principles underlying WHO's public health approach to ART, including standardised, simplified, low-cost quality assured treatment regimens, decentralised and integrated healthcare services and free care at the point of delivery are carefully explored in this book. Approaches successfully applied to HIV, and now across multiple health challenges, include support to meaningful community engagement and leveraging multisectoral policy and action as part of broader efforts to ensure that sustainable and equitable health systems are built to reach the most vulnerable and marginalised populations.

WHO's public health approach for other communicable and non-communicable diseases (NCDs) builds on the valuable lessons and strategies learned from four decades of work on HIV that can be applied to their control and prevention. The authors examine the successes, challenges and adaptations required to optimally apply this approach to NCDs, considering the unique nature of these diseases and their risk factors.

As nations strive to address increasingly complex global health challenges, it becomes increasingly important to adopt holistic people-centred approaches that prioritise the health and well-being of individuals, communities and populations.

Most of the world continues to lack access to quality essential health services and inequalities persist, driving WHO's focus on universal health coverage. WHO recognises that the primary healthcare approach, with its focus on providing essential primary care services, community engagement and multisectoral policy and action as central to efforts towards achieving universal health coverage.

The authors present the transformative potential of this approach and its ability to address the health needs of diverse communities emphasising the importance of health systems strengthening, primary health care and financial protection mechanisms. The synergy between these elements is crucial for the development of effective and efficient health systems that guarantee the provision of quality services for all.

This book is a useful reference in our collective journey towards health for all. It serves as a valuable resource for policymakers, healthcare practitioners, researchers and students by offering insights, best practices and practical recommendations for the implementation of this approach in different contexts.

I encourage all students to delve into the pages of this book and engage in the critical discussions it presents. Together, let us recognise the potential of the WHO's public health approach in transforming systems for health to ensure health and promote well-being worldwide. By widely embracing it, we can move closer to the realisation of UHC and a world where no one is left behind.

Dr Tedros Adhanom Ghebreyesus
Director-General, World Health Organization

Preface

Drawing on their background in HIV/AIDS and global public health, the authors aim to describe how the staggering successes in HIV/AIDS control over the last two decades has come about; and then consider what this can and should mean for two of the pressing health challenges facing the global south today – controlling and coping with the epidemic of chronic non-communicable diseases and progressing universal health coverage particularly for those most at risk of financial hardship.

The book has three sections which cover HIV/AIDS, the chronic NCDs and UHC. Each considers equity and human rights and broadly follows a common format: a description of the health challenge; an outline of global commitments to action made at the UN by member states, WHO and others; a review of the steps taken to dealing with the health issue; a brief note on the impact of the SARS-CoV-2/COVID-19 pandemic; and an analysis of the successes achieved and challenges that still remain for achieving the Sustainable Development Goals targets for 2030 and beyond.

Section 1 also details the WHO public health approach to ART and HIV/AIDS control: how it came about to address global inequity in access to treatment and care; and how through the "3by5" intervention, strategic thinking was turned into programmatic action and realisable outcomes. It outlines how the public health approach has been updated and kept fit for purpose to sustainably increase access to ART and treatment coverage globally such that HIV is now endemic and AIDS is on track to end in most countries by 2030.

Section 2 also highlights that while the NCDs are increasingly important, they remain neglected and in crisis. It asks why; and considers how the public health approach could be adopted and adapted to the NCDs and other disease control priorities in resource-limited settings to help scale up relevant control interventions. Pivoting to integrated service delivery this supports quality care and facilitates health systems strengthening at the primary care level linked with the district hospital.

Section 3 also looks at progress made and challenges remaining for universal health coverage, considering health services, financial risk protection, out-of-pocket health spending, impoverishment and catastrophic health spending. It outlines specific ways in which public health approaches can be deployed towards UHC by integrating a range of strategies encompassing health, disease prevention and equitable access to quality services through strengthened health systems and by addressing the social, economic and environmental determinants of health.

The subject matter in the book is broad but should interest a wide variety of stakeholders involved in global public health including students, academics, health practitioners, planners and policymakers, development experts, donors and national decision-makers. Asking why ART scale-up was successful and how the public health approach, the key to that success can readily be applied to the NCDs and then drive progress towards UHC is novel. The key thesis that significant practical progress can be made and health systems strengthened by an integrated public health approach is relevant to all.

Acknowledgements

Writing a book is always a team effort, and ours is no exception. Over the course of developing the concept and then writing our book we have drawn on the advice and support of many colleagues with whom we have had the privilege of working closely with and learning from over the years at the University of Queensland, Addis Ababa University, Imperial College London, the Institute of Tropical Medicine in Antwerp, Oxford University, the Liverpool School of Tropical Medicine and the Ethiopian Public Health Institute.

We have learned much from exceptional colleagues, dedicated development specialists and health professionals in the UK Department for International Development. We have over the years been privileged to work with and learn much from some exceptional individuals in the UN and particularly in three agencies – WHO, UNICEF and UNAIDS; and at country level in Ethiopia particularly in the Ministry of Health as well as health providers in India, Kenya, Uganda and Malawi. Among many, a special mention needs to be given to Marleen Boelart, Siobhan Crowley, Janet Darbyshire, Neil French, Haileye-sus Getahun, Damen Hailemariam, Marie Laga, Julian Lob-Levyt, Lut Lynen, Philip Marsden, Pete McDermot, Paula Munderi, David Nabarro, Peter Piot, Marjan Pirard, Carole Presern, Marco Vitoria, David Warrell and Jon Weber.

All of our work has been grounded by the lived experiences of people living with HIV and community leaders who have aimed to make a difference. We have been inspired by their strength, activism and dedication to improving access to ART as a human right to all in need regardless of the ability to pay. We particularly recognise the contributions of Zachie Achmet, Gregg Gonsalves, Mark Harrington and Noerine Kaleeba. From these interactions, we have deeply appreciated the challenges of disease control and healthcare delivery in settings with limited resources and capacity; and the need to support universal access to ART by developing and delivering the public health approach to HIV/AIDS.

There are several people who we need to single out to and specifically thank for their support and inputs as we have pondered what the lessons for the NCDs and UHC are from the successes with implementing a WHO public health approach to HIV/AIDS and put the book together: Peter Hill, Simon Reid and Chris Shannon at UQ; Wim Van Damme in Antwerp; and Stephen Moses in Canada.

We thank our students who have always encouraged us in our project and dealt with our stresses and pressures; and give a special thanks to Aklilu Endalamaw and Resham Khatri. Russell George, our senior editor in Routledge, has been patient and very helpful as our book has slowly come together and we thank him for his encouragement and support.

Finally special thanks to Marina and Blen and our families who have put up with a lot but always been there as our book has evolved and gestated and finally been published. They have asked incisive questions, made helpful suggestions and constantly encouraged us. They are looking forward to the new post-book normal and are relieved our project has successfully come to an end.

Abbreviations and acronyms

ACE	Angiotensin-converting-enzyme, inhibitors of which control blood pressure
ACP	AIDS Control Programme
ACT UP	The AIDS Coalition to Unleash Power
AIDS	Acquired immunodeficiency (immune deficiency) syndrome
AMDS	AIDS Medicines and Diagnostics Service
AMR	Antimicrobial resistance
ART	Antiretroviral therapy/treatment
ARV	Antiretroviral, medicines used for HIV treatment
AZT	Zidovudine, an antiretroviral medicine in the NRTI class
BMI	Body-mass index, an assessment of weight and obesity
BP	Blood pressure; when raised is often referred to as hypertension
CAB	Cabotegravir, an antiretroviral medicine in the Capsid Inhibitor class
CAB-LA	Long-acting injectable cabotegravir
CBHI	Community-based health insurance
CDC	Centers for Disease Control, now Centers for Disease Control and Prevention, USA
CEA	Cost-effectiveness analysis
CIs	Confidence intervals around an estimate, usually at the 95% level
CKD	Chronic kidney disease
COPD	Chronic obstructive pulmonary disease
COVID-19	The disease manifestations of SARS-CoV-2 infection
CRD	Chronic respiratory diseases
CTX	Co-trimoxazole, used as prophylaxis to prevent opportunistic infections
CVD	Cardiovascular disease

DAH	Development Assistance for Health, from bilateral and multilateral donor sources
DALY	Disability-adjusted life-years
DCP	Disease Control Priorities referring to those in developing countries
DCP1,2,3	The various editions of the Disease Control Priority books
DG	Director-General (usually of WHO)
DH	Digital Health
DPV	Dapivirine, an antiretroviral medicine in the NNRTI class
DSD	Differentiated service delivery
EBP	Essential Benefits Package
ECG	Electrocardiograph, a test to assess heart function and rhythm
EHSBP	Essential Health Services Benefits Plan
EIA	Enzyme ImmunoAssay, a type of laboratory test, also known as an ELISA test
EPI	Expanded Programme on Immunisation
EUHC	Essential Universal Health Coverage
ET	Epidemiological Transition
FCTC	The Framework Convention on Tobacco Control, a WHO initiative
FSW	Female sex worker
G8	Group of Eight intergovernmental political forum 1997–2014; now G7
GAP	WHO's Global Action Plan for NCD prevention and control
GAVI	Global Alliance for Vaccines and Immunisation now Gavi, the Vaccine Alliance
GBD	Global Burden of Disease
GFATM	The Global Fund to fight AIDS, Tuberculosis and Malaria; or simply the Global Fund
GHI	Global Health Initiative
GHS	Global Health Security
GIPA	Greater involvement of People with AIDS
GMHC	Gay Men's Health Crisis
HBV	Hepatitis B virus
HCV	Hepatitis C virus
HIV	Human immunodeficiency virus
HIVDR	HIV drug resistance
HIVST	HIV self-testing
HLM	High Level Meeting (of the UN General Assembly)
HPV	Human papilloma virus
HSS	Health System Strengthening
HTS	HIV testing services

ICD	International Classification of Disease
IDU	Injecting drug user
IMAI/IMCI	Integrated Management of Adult or Childhood Illness
IHR	International Health Regulations set by WHO to control transboundary infections
IMSS	Instituto Mexicano del Seguro Social, Mexico's healthcare system
INSTIs	Integrase Strand Transfer/Integrase Inhibitors, a class of ARV medicines
IPCHS	Integrated People-centred Health Services
IPT	Isoniazid preventive therapy, prophylaxis for TB
LA	Long-acting, in respect of ARV formulations with a long duration of action
LMIC	Low- and middle-income countries
MABs	Monoclonal antibodies, used for HIV immunotherapy
MCH/MNCH	Maternal and Child Health services, often now including Newborn services
MDGs	Millennium development goals
MI	Myocardial infarction, commonly referred to as heart attack
MSM	Men who have sex with men
NCDs	Non-communicable diseases
NGO	Non-government organisation
NHIS	National Health Insurance Scheme
NHS	National Health Service, the UK public health system
NNRTIs	Non-nucleoside reverse transcriptase Inhibitors, a class of ARV medicines
NRT	Nicotine replacement therapy, for smoking cessation
NRTIs	Nucleoside(tide) reverse transcriptase inhibitors, a class of ARV medicines
NTDs	Neglected tropical diseases
OIs	Opportunistic infections
OOP	Out-of-pocket, for payment for services
PEN	Package of Essential Non-communicable disease interventions, a WHO initiative
PEP	Post exposure prophylaxis for HIV
PEPFAR	The United States President's Emergency Plan for AIDS Relief
PHC	Primary Healthcare
PHEIC	Public Health Emergency of International Concern
PITC	Provider initiated HIV testing and counselling
PIs	Protease inhibitors, a class of ARV medicines
PLHA	Person/people living with HIV/AIDS
PLHIV	Person/people living with HIV

PLWNCD	People living with non-communicable diseases
PMTCT	Prevention of mother to child transmission of HIV
POC	Point-of-care
PrEP	Pre-exposure prophylaxis for HIV
RDT	Rapid diagnostic test
RPV	Rilpivirine, an antiretroviral medicine in the NNRTI class
SARS-CoV-2	The coronavirus that causes COVID-19 disease
SC	Security Council (of the United Nations)
SCI	Service Coverage Index, to monitor UHC service coverage
SDGs	Sustainable development goals
SDH	Social Determinants of Health
SSA	Sub-saharan Africa
T&T	Test and Treat (for HIV)
TAC	Treatment Action Campaign
TAG	Treatment Action Group
TASO	The AIDS Support Organization
TB	Tuberculosis
TDF	Tenofovir, an antiretroviral medicine in the NRTI class
TLD	Tenofovir-Lamivudine-Darunavir, a widely used first-line co-formulated medicine
TLE	Tenofovir-Lamivudine-Efavirenz, a widely used first-line co-formulated medicine
TRIPS	Trade-Related Aspects of Intellectual Property Rights
U=U	Undetectable (viral load) = Untransmissible (HIV infection)
UHC	Universal health coverage
UHSC	Universal health services coverage
UN	United Nations
UNAIDS	Joint United Nations Programme on HIV/AIDS (UNAIDS)
UNGASS	UN General Assembly Special Session
US/USA	United States
VCT	Voluntary testing and counselling (for HIV)
WHA	World Health Assembly
WHO	World Health Organization

Introduction

Setting the context

At the turn of the millennium human immunodeficiency virus (HIV) was spreading rapidly across the world and millions were becoming infected from a preventable but readily transmissible infection. Most went on to die prematurely with acquired immunodeficiency syndrome (AIDS), a constellation of opportunistic diseases and cancers that were a direct consequence of uncontrolled viral replication and the insidious slow destruction of the immune system. Stigma and discrimination were widespread; some countries were close to collapse. The United Nations (UN) Security Council declared HIV/AIDS a security issue that if unchecked posed a grave risk to global stability.

There was a glimmer of hope: effective medicines had been developed and antiretroviral therapy (ART) was beginning to revolutionise AIDS care and disease outcome, transforming it from a death sentence to a chronic, incurable disease. ART was generally available and widely used in high-income countries that could afford it; and that had robust, well-equipped healthcare services with specialist physicians who could provide quality services and manage complex treatment regimens.

The main burden of disease was however in the global south and particularly in sub-Saharan Africa, which was bearing the brunt of the AIDS epidemic. There was a huge treatment gap: costly ART was unavailable in public sector health services; poorly-equipped hospitals were being overwhelmed by sick and dying patients with AIDS. The UN General Assembly made closing the treatment gap a global health priority; HIV/AIDS figured prominently in the Millennium Development Goals, with a specific target to achieve by 2010 universal access to treatment for all who needed it.

Most thought this was impossible and that treatment would never be widely available across the global south. However, slowly but surely the treatment gap has been closed. ART coverage now exceeds 75% and is still rising; many believe that we are well on track to achieve the sustainable development goals (SDGs) target to end AIDS as a public health threat by 2030.

DOI: 10.4324/9781003505693-1

Enabling almost all individuals living with HIV in resource-limited settings to access life-saving ART according to need rather than affordability and the ability to pay is a remarkable achievement. It is already widely regarded as one of the main global public health triumphs of the first two decades of the 21st century. Such progress has not been seen in other disease control programmes.

There is an extensive literature on the HIV epidemic and the successful approaches AIDS control programmes in the global south have adopted. However little has been written on how ART has been scaled up so dramatically and successfully against all expectation. And no consideration of how these achievements could be replicated to combat other pressing disease control priorities, in particular the epidemic non-communicable diseases (NCDs); or what this could mean for driving forward the universal health coverage (UHC) agenda. This book seeks to fill this void.

As will be clear in the first section of the book, the World Health Organisation (WHO) public health approach to ART was pivotal in closing the treatment gap and sustaining treatment and prevention scale-up over the last two decades. The second section considers how a similar simplified and standardised public health approach could be developed for the complex chronic NCDs; and then delivered in ways that strengthen primary healthcare and primary care services within a capacitated district health team and integrated with the district hospital. The last section of the book considers how a more complete range of essential services using the public health approach and delivered through greatly strengthened health systems can drive UHC; and give countries the confidence to scale up the necessary investments to achieve this.

Conceptualising a public health approach

Highly effective ART to treat HIV infection was developed remarkably rapidly in the global north, particularly in the United States of America (USA). It was arguably the most important tangible product of the unprecedented response to the epidemic that had started almost as soon as AIDS was recognised and first described in 1981. At the onset, there was widespread fear of the unknown, and concern that everyone could be at risk from the potentially unstoppable spread of this new plague.

With strong and vocal civil society activism, including many who were living with HIV and sick with AIDS, there was a growing consensus that something needed to be done, and fast, to combat the epidemic. It soon became generally accepted that AIDS required an exceptional response above and beyond normal health interventions to protect the rights of those at special risk, to generate resources to assist affected communities and sufficient to control the then mysterious epidemic.

Huge ring-fenced investments were made into research towards a vaccine and effective medicines. Civil society activists transcended the hateful views of the moral majority that the gay community, sex workers and injecting drug users were bringing this on themselves; and generated strong bipartisan political commitment for wide access to care support and treatment regardless of the ability to pay. By the turn of the millennium, combination therapy transformed AIDS from a death sentence to a treatable chronic disease. But ART was very costly and extremely complex to use.

These developments were happening as it was slowly being realised that HIV and AIDS was widely spread around the globe. The advances in AIDS care and treatment were largely by-passing low- and middle-income countries that could not afford to provide ART in the public health sector, which was itself largely without the sophisticated medical technology and cadres of specialist physicians who were regarded as indispensable for its delivery. Such global inequity was troubling many, and there were growing voices for ART to be made widely available to those who needed it. The UN, member states, civil society and people living with HIV/AIDS (PLHA) were united in calling for the treatment gap to be closed as a global health priority. This would however require a massive scale-up of service provision and drug supply. And the belief that it could be effectively delivered.

Treatment scale-up of this magnitude across the global south was viewed by some global health experts as a futile exercise and by others as mission impossible. There was concern that widescale ART provision was unaffordable; and if embarked upon would distort development budgets and compromise other critical public health and nutrition programmes. Many were sceptical about an overt clinical and biomedical approach focussing on ART; prevention should continue to be centre-stage and the mainstay of all AIDS Control Programmes. It was often claimed that we couldn't treat our way out of the epidemic; some believed we shouldn't even try.

Downplaying or ignoring the pressing care, support and treatment needs of millions of individuals in resource-limited settings did not chime well with people living with HIV/AIDS, nor with civil society that was concerned with social justice. Health was increasingly regarded as a key human rights issue: with a rights-based approach, it became generally accepted that access to ART was a fundamental element of the right of all people to the enjoyment of the highest attainable standard of health.

With the continuing rollout of more potent, less toxic treatment in rich industrialised settings, it was time to broaden AIDS exceptionalism to the global stage and ensure that treatment programmes were properly funded in resource-constrained settings. Politicians of all shades were persuaded that something had to be done as a priority to address the treatment gap. New financing mechanisms were established which rapidly resulted in significant new resources being allocated for ART rollout; aspirational goals and ambitious targets for ART rollout were set.

Whilst necessary, new resources by themselves were insufficient without a clear plan of action on how antiretroviral medicines could effectively be deployed in resource-constrained settings with limited health infrastructure and capacity, a dearth of specialist physicians and insufficient human resources for health. The concept of a public health approach was developed in WHO to overcome these challenges and to make ART accessible to all in need. Global guidelines with clear protocols were produced by WHO then regularly updated to guide HIV diagnosis, biomedical prevention, AIDS care and treatment in populations accessing healthcare in the public sector.

Looking back, it is remarkable that such strong interest was given to closing the treatment gap and addressing the stark inequity in AIDS deaths between rich industrialised countries and sub-Saharan Africa. There had been limited progress with primary healthcare and the attainment of better health for all since the landmark 1978 Declaration of Alma-Ata. Other longstanding disparities in nutrition, family planning access, maternal mortality, health status, disability and disease outcome had failed to attract attention or clarion calls for action. Apart from child survival and the Children's Vaccine Initiative (then GAVI, now Gavi, the Vaccine Alliance) launched in 1990, there had been no special commitment to mobilise the resources necessary to have significant impact.

The speed with which new international (Global Fund) and bilateral (President's Emergency Plan for AIDS Relief) funding mechanisms were established in response to an acknowledged global health emergency is also quite remarkable. Joining GAVI, it is notable that all three major Global Health Initiatives (GHIs) raise and disburse additional funds for infectious disease treatment and control. It has taken nearly 30 years for a new UN fund for loss and damage due to climate change to emerge from the UN Climate Change Conference COP27 in 2022: the initial idea for such a fund was first floated by Vanuatu in 1991. The very rapid response to the SARS-CoV-2/COVID-19 pandemic, across diagnostics, vaccines, care and therapeutics, came from the pharmaceutical sector or national clinical research bodies; it did not need to wait for global funding mechanisms.

As it unfolded, the global response has been maintained and sustained. WHO leadership proved crucial: with wide availability of antiretroviral medicines, there has been massive expansion of biomedical prevention. Additional resources have been invested even as substantial annual programme costs increase year on year. The public health approach to ART has evolved and remained the central pillar and mainstay of treatment scale-up and biomedical prevention in the global south. The global community is on track to deliver on the SDG target to end the epidemic of AIDS as a public health threat by 2030.

Such success in ART scale-up, and by extension with biomedical prevention, has been achieved within the context of a vertical programme and with considerable global AIDS exceptionalism. Population health needs are evolving even as HIV/AIDS is better prevented and treated. With the epidemiological transition and a changing burden of disease in low- and middle-income countries, other health priorities are coming to the fore and competing for limited resources for health within a constrained funding envelope.

Looking to the future, without an effective vaccine or cure more will have to be done with less, as we strive to realise the global goal of ending AIDS as a public health problem by 2030. Services will increasingly need to be integrated at the primary care level and linked with hospital care across the district health team as disease control programmes for NCDs are ramped up. The public health approach will remain central. Building on the key elements of success is vital: what has worked; how horizontal integration is best delivered and health systems are strengthened; what can be done more efficiently without compromising service quality; how primary healthcare is best promoted.

Beyond HIV/AIDS towards other complex chronic diseases

By itself, the story behind the public health triumph of ART scale-up merits the publication of a specialist monograph. Few would think it substantial enough to justify a stand-alone textbook or companion handbook: the subject matter would most likely be of interest only to those involved in HIV/AIDS control in the global south. Most such practitioners are already familiar with the genesis of the public health approach; how it has been implemented to great effect and evolved over time to remain fit for purpose; and are very aware of the remaining challenges particularly needing to do more with less. Learning from the successes to date and translating this to overcoming current and future challenges is important but would only have a relatively small audience/readership.

The book aims to go beyond HIV/AIDS to consider how lessons learnt in developing then deploying the public health approach over the last two decades in one vertical programme are relevant to and could easily be adapted and adopted by other priority disease control programmes in low- and middle-income countries. The approaches used to simplify and standardise diagnostic pathways, to support entry and retention in care services and extend management protocols out to the primary care level are broadly applicable. Delivering medicine at scale allows so much to be achieved in reducing morbidity and mortality and through biomedical prevention.

Non-communicable diseases kill over 40 million people each year, equivalent to at least 70% of all deaths globally. They disproportionately affect people in low- and middle-income countries where more than three quarters of global NCD deaths occur: most are considered premature occurring between the ages of 30 and 69. Four groups of diseases account for almost all premature NCD deaths: cardiovascular diseases (such as heart attacks and stroke); cancers; chronic respiratory diseases (such as asthma and chronic obstructive pulmonary disease) and diabetes.

The UN has for many years recognised NCDs as a major public health challenge. WHO's World Health Report 2002 "Reducing risks, promoting healthy life" drew attention to the importance of what were then called chronic diseases and their contribution to the global burden of disease. The 64th session of the UN

General Assembly in 2010 resolved to encourage UN member states to address the issue of NCDs. The SDGs adopted by the UN in 2015 included the NCDs with a specific target to reduce premature NCD mortality by one-third by 2030.

The NCDs have largely failed to become a focus for activism and target-driven public health with few pressure groups urging action, pushing for more appropriate resource allocation and better disease control programmes: there is no exceptional NCD response or new funding mechanisms for chronic diseases. The cumbersome NCD construct and the limited public understanding of the importance of the agenda may play a part; as may the complexities and challenges in implementing prevention policy and disease management interventions to effectively control them. Another constraint may be the multiplicity of programmes needed for each NCD, without common themes or opportunities for integrated service delivery. It seems too difficult a task.

The most recent 2022 WHO NCD Progress monitor notes limited progress and missed opportunities and finds that simple and effective interventions are not being adopted widely enough around the world to impact the NCD pandemic and reduce morbidity and mortality. While politicians and donor agencies are aware of the changing burden of disease and their growing importance, limited new funds are available to support countries or communities to develop effective policy and programmes to impact NCD mortality. This starkly contrasts with the achievements in closing the AIDS treatment gap over the same decades: much can be learned from successful scale-up and HIV/AIDS control.

New thinking and new approaches are needed. One key step is to transcend the communicable/non-communicable binary that separates the chronic NCDs from transmissible HIV/AIDS. Both HIV/AIDS and the individual NCDs are complex to prevent with an array of policy interventions, biobehavioural and biomedical interventions; and seemingly complex to treat because they are without a cure, so following diagnosis, care support and treatment is lifelong and without an obvious endpoint.

Focussing on the differences, failing to see the similarities deters planners and policymakers from appreciating and critically evaluating the clear lessons from successful ART scale-up. It inadvertently obscures the similar spread of health service activities from screening and diagnosis then entry into a care programme and embarking upon a treatment pathway that includes biomedical prevention. It inhibits the development and implementation of a new public health approach to NCDs.

Focussing on the similarities, the health system synergies between HIV/AIDS and NCDs would be better recognised; the development of integrated service delivery models especially at the primary care level and across the district health team would permit improved disease outcome across both challenges. The belief that effective interventions can be delivered using a public health approach can be fostered. If it can be done for HIV/AIDS, it can and should be done for the chronic NCDs.

The public health approach to ART embodies the essential values of PHC in the Declaration of Alma-Ata – social justice and the right to better health for all, participation and solidarity. All the specific elements were developed for use in public sector health services financed by the state. The focus was on population rather than individual-level clinical guidance down to the primary care level. These values and elements are critical to address the NCD crisis and the stalled agenda.

Building on the increasing recognition in many quarters of the importance of the chronic NCDs and the need for more appropriate resource allocation to achieve better health outcomes and reduce morbidity and mortality, it is time that the same public health approach lens is turned on diabetes, cardiovascular disease and other NCDs. Like HIV/AIDS they are complex to treat and control at the primary care level; and are incurable requiring lifelong service delivery that seems hugely challenging to sustain at the population level.

This is the key thesis in the second section of the book – to imagine how the development and implementation of the public health approach for HIV/AIDS can be adopted, adapted and applied to the NCDs. It can simply be broadened out to cover mental health, not currently included in the NCD portfolio; and by promoting health system strengthening can encompass other disease control priorities that are major contributors to morbidity and premature mortality across the global south.

The ultimate challenge: securing universal health coverage

Universal health coverage (UHC) is the radical, for some, proposition that everyone should have equitable access to the high-quality health services they need without suffering financial hardship. It includes the full spectrum of essential, quality health services from health promotion to prevention, treatment, rehabilitation and palliative care across the life course. The delivery of these services requires adequate and competent health professionals with optimal skills mix at facility, outreach and community level, who are equitably distributed, adequately supported and enjoy decent work conditions. It requires significant new resources and much additional funding for health devoted to health system strengthening rather than vertical disease control programmes.

The need for UHC is clear. Half the world's population do not have access to the healthcare they need. When households have to pay most of the costs for health services out of their own pockets, the poor are often unable to obtain many of the services they need; and even the rich may be exposed to financial hardship in the event of severe or chronic long-term illness. Each year, it is estimated that 100 million people are driven into poverty through out-of-pocket health spending.

UHC policies and strategies enable everyone to access the prevention and care services they need to address the most significant causes of disease and death; and ensures that the quality of those services is good enough to improve the health of the people and communities who receive them. To cover all ages and different needs a life-course approach is mandated. Primary healthcare is the base for, and the most important pathway to achieve UHC. It could be argued that UHC has now become the roadmap towards the objective of WHO when it was founded in 1948: the highest attainable standard of health for all people.

Achieving UHC requires multiple approaches and a fundamental shift in service delivery such that health interventions are integrated and focus on the needs of people and communities. Improving the quality of healthcare, health service coverage and health outcomes depend on the availability, accessibility and capacity of healthcare workers to deliver quality people-centred integrated care. Properly maintained, well-stocked and accessible health facilities are essential, particularly at the primary care and community level. Robust financing structures are key. Without proper resourcing, UHC will remain an aspirational goal, a great concept but unrealisable, impractical and unachievable in the poorest countries and communities most in need of it.

High-level political engagement and multilateral buy-in are critical. Since the 2001 WHO Commission on Macroeconomics and Health, good health has been recognised as essential to sustainable economic development: invest substantially in health and economic development will follow. The third SDG focusses on good health and well-being, aiming to ensure healthy lives and promote well-being for all at all ages: target 3.8 is to achieve UHC, including financial risk prevention, access to quality essential healthcare services and access to safe, effective, quality and affordable essential medicines and vaccines for all.

Progress has been patchy in those countries and regions of the world that report on UHC. The 2019 UHC Global Monitoring Report (prepared by WHO, the World Bank and the OECD) had some stark messages. If current trends continue up to 5 billion people will still be unable to access healthcare in 2030; impoverishment due to paying for healthcare increased except among the very poor. About 925 million people spent more than 10%, 200 million more than 25% of income on healthcare. The world will need to increase health coverage and improve care quality to achieve UHC with more urgency now as we emerge from the SARS-CoV-2/COVID-19 pandemic.

To meet 2030 targets, over 18 million additional health workers will be required, mainly in the global south. WHO recommends that every country allocate or reallocate an additional 1% of GDP to PHC from government and external funding sources. Scaling up quality interventions across low- and middle-income countries could have a massive impact and save 60 million lives and increase life expectancy by 3.7 years by 2030. But will it? Beyond taking on more health professionals and greatly increasing health financing there is little practical detail in UHC policy to suggest what exactly to do with these precious resources to ensure improved health and well-being, better treatment outcomes and less household health expenditure. As always, the devil is in the detail.

The public health approach, as we suggest in the book, can readily be applied to the NCDs and other disease control priorities across the life-course with considerable impact and benefit. Effectively integrating these services at the primary care level with a special focus on logistics and common supply chains will enhance access to and use of essential medicines, contraceptives for family planning and vaccines for full childhood immunisations. Strengthening the hub and spoke clinic and hospital service delivery unit in line with the public health approach through harmonised care guidelines and task-shifting will increase basic hospital access when referrals up and down are made within simple standard care pathways. In fact, almost all the essential healthcare services that are included in the WHO framework as indicators to monitor progress towards UHC can be strongly and positively impacted by the general use and adoption of a public health approach.

Quality HIV services can be taken to scale and financial hardship minimised. Knowing that the public health approach that made this happen is readily applicable to the NCDs and other disease control priorities should give finance ministers in the global south, and bilateral donors and multilateral funding bodies high confidence to invest in UHC. Health worker density will increase as and when more finances are raised for UHC, particularly to recruit and retain health workers at the primary care level where they are most lacking. With better outcomes across the burden of disease (rather than a few donor priorities) will encourage more investment in UHC: a virtuous circle is created.

Securing UHC is the ultimate challenge in ensuring the highest attainable standard of health for all people. The last section of the book considers how a more complete range of essential services using the public health approach based on a life course approach and integrated at the primary healthcare level is entirely practical in design and feasible to implement; and will rapidly make a significant contribution to poverty alleviation and achieving UHC.

Using this book to best effect

We intend that our book will interest a wide variety of stakeholders involved in global public health, from students and academics, clinicians and health practitioners, planners and policymakers, to development specialists, donors and national decision-makers. With such a broad and diverse target audience with different levels of experience and expertise, the book can variously be considered as a research monograph, a textbook or even a handbook or companion; and can be used in different ways to suit the reader's needs and expectations.

The subject matter is broad but does cover a far-reaching cross-section of contemporary global public health issues: the essential values of primary healthcare; health systems strengthening and vertical disease control programming; the importance of integrated service delivery; how success in HIV/AIDS with the WHO public health approach could translate to other priority health areas. It considers the two most pressing health and development challenges of the next 30 years – the epidemic of NCDs and the need to make heavy investments in health to achieve UHC. Uniquely the book gives hope that progress can be made in these critical areas where much has been discussed at the policy level, but little delivered at the practical level, particularly but not just in the global south.

Asking why ART scale-up was successful and how the public health approach, the key to that success, can readily be applied to other complex chronic NCDs and then drive progress towards UHC is novel. The message that significant practical progress can be made in combating NCDs following a tried and tested approach in ART scale-up and HIV/AIDS control is timely and important, given the limited progress made to date. The fact that appropriately resourcing one disease control priority area can successfully deliver quality services to most in need without financial hardship should encourage the substantial new investments in health and help drive progress to secure UHC.

From the student perspective, using the example of HIV/AIDS control and treatment scale-up well illustrates how advocacy moves agendas and influences funding allocation, how a very successful disease control programme can be built from scratch, and how the public health approach is the cornerstone of effectively translating policy into practice. It outlines the NCD agenda, the challenges and potential ways to control them. It outlines the UHC agenda and how this can be advanced.

For global health academics, the challenge is getting research into policy and practice to equitably improve health and well-being. This closely links with implementation science, the study of methods and strategies that facilitate the uptake of evidence-based practice and research into regular use by practitioners and policymakers. We believe there will be food for thought in our book, particularly in health sector strengthening and service integration; and developing new approaches to progress NCD delivery and securing UHC.

For clinicians and health professionals involved in the prevention and treatment of communicable and chronic NCDs and the planners and policymakers involved in design and implementation, it is important to understand the drivers of the shift away from vertical towards more horizontal disease control programmes; and the centrality of the district health team to support integrated service delivery. And to fully recognise and appreciate the benefits of a practical public health approach across the life course to enable this to improve NCD care and services towards UHC.

Development specialists, donors and national decision-makers aim to improve health and well-being, by impacting the NCD epidemic and making tangible progress towards UHC while sustaining the successes achieved with HIV/AIDS control. The expectation is that our core thesis, the need to incorporate the practical public health approach in disease control programming to drive better service integration, will be a refreshing contribution to policy development and implementation; and will give confidence for new investments in health systems strengthening to be made.

Section 1

The WHO public health approach to HIV/AIDS in the global south

1 Recognising and addressing inequity in the global HIV/ AIDS response

Human immunodeficiency virus and acquired immunodeficiency syndrome

Human immunodeficiency virus (HIV) types 1 and 2 are zoonotic retroviruses that have frequently crossed over into human populations from monkeys and apes that are the natural hosts for several simian counterpart retroviruses and are enzootic in West and Central Africa. HIV usually refers to type 1 infection which globally predominates as the cause of acquired immunodeficiency syndrome (AIDS); type 2 is restricted to West Africa. HIV became epidemic in the 1950s and 1960s in Africa then crossed into the Americas, and soon became pandemic. The story of the early years of the HIV/AIDS epidemic is well told by Jacques Pepin in his book, *The Origins of AIDS* (Pepin, 2011).

HIV is highly pathogenic in humans: over months and years, the virus replicates in CD4 lymphocytes and slowly destroys the integrity of the immune system. This renders the infected individual more susceptible to certain unusual diseases – some rare cancers and several characteristic opportunistic infections (OIs). When clusters of these unusual diseases were first reported in the United States in 1981, in individuals with no obvious reason to be immunodeficient, the centres for disease control (CDC) created a case definition for surveillance purposes of several OIs and cancers characteristic of severe immunosuppression and a name was given to this emerging problem: AIDS. The World Health Organization (WHO) adopted the CDC case definition in 1986 for global AIDS surveillance purposes (World Health Organization (WHO), 1986). In common parlance, the acronym AIDS is now taken to mean severe and usually fatal disease consequent on HIV infection, in the same way that SARS-CoV-2 is the virus that causes COVID-19 disease.

AIDS surveillance in the United States rapidly revealed a fast-growing epidemic of uncertain cause, clustering in some at-risk groups but also occurring sporadically. At the onset, there was widespread fear of the unknown, and concern that everyone could be at risk from the potentially unstoppable spread of

DOI: 10.4324/9781003505693-3

this new lethal plague. The race was on to identify the cause of this deadly epidemic. By 1983, a new retrovirus eventually called HIV was isolated from a French patient with AIDS-related complex in France (Barré-Sinoussi et al., 1983). Professors Francoise Barre-Sinoussi and Luc Montanier were awarded the 2008 Nobel Prize for their discovery.

Finding a virus was the crucial first step to develop reliable and accurate serological tests for both patient diagnosis and epidemiological studies, and to understand its pathogenesis. As a blood-borne virus (BBV) HIV is present in blood and anogenital secretions: it is transmitted sexually, from mother to child (in utero, during birth and via breast milk) and via blood transfusion. Gay and bisexual men who have sex with men (MSM) and injection drug users (IDU) are particularly vulnerable: these risk groups predominate in high-income settings; countries experience a concentrated HIV epidemic. Global surveillance soon revealed that HIV was becoming pandemic and was particularly prevalent in sub-Saharan Africa where heterosexual sex was the predominant transmission route: in generalised epidemics, men, women and children are infected and female sex workers are highly vulnerable.

With significant stigma and discrimination (including unfortunately from healthcare professionals) patients were counselled pre-test and if diagnosed with HIV offered supportive post-test counselling. As the AIDS epidemic progressed, the initial care, support and treatment interventions for person/people living with HIV/AIDS (PLHAs) were relatively restricted to prevention and treatment of HIV-related OIs and cancers, counselling and psychosocial support and palliative care. Community-based organisations took on much of the care and support burden: home-based care was important, with family members, PLHA and buddies from the community supporting the sick and dying.

With strong and vocal civil society activism in the global north, including many who were living with HIV and sick with AIDS, there was a growing consensus that something needed to be done, and fast, to combat the epidemic. It soon became generally accepted that AIDS required an exceptional response above and beyond normal health interventions to protect the rights of those at special risk, to generate resources to assist affected communities and sufficient to control the then mysterious AIDS epidemic (Smith & Whiteside, 2010).

Huge, ring-fenced investments were made to fast-track research to develop diagnostics, vaccines and therapeutics. While there is still no effective vaccine for HIV, nor have effective cure strategies yet been developed, unprecedented progress has been made in the development of highly accurate diagnostics, including point-of-care (POC) devices that are particularly suitable for resource-limited settings and for HIV self-testing (Manoto et al., 2018); and in developing several different classes of highly effective antiretroviral medicines for both treatment and prevention of HIV infection.

Global political commitments and policy setting to close the treatment gap

Global inequity in access to HIV/AIDS services, in particular ART, and gross disparities in disease outcome and survival, were troubling many at the turn of the millennium. Before this, starting in the United States, vocal PLHA activist groups and community support organisations sprung up: civil society activists started to challenge the hateful views of the moral majority that the gay community, sex workers and injecting drug users were bringing AIDS on themselves. Over time, they generated bipartisan political commitment for wide access to care and support, and ART when it was available, regardless of the ability to pay. With their experience and community engagement, they were to become strong partners in advocacy, guideline development and ART delivery.

The greater involvement of people with HIV/AIDS (GIPA) was particularly important: protest and survive; nothing about us without us. For the first time, people with infection or disease were consulted and involved in care and service delivery: the patient perspective became an important consideration for planners and policymakers. In a fast-moving field, well-informed patients often knew as much if not more than their specialist physicians (Morolake et al., 2009).

Across the global south, National AIDS Control Programmes with civil society organisations, brave PLHA activists, public health practitioners, specialist physicians, scientists and researchers with significant support from bilateral and multilateral development agencies started intensively to focus on ways that these grave inequities could be addressed, and in particular how the growing "treatment gap" could be overcome. Remarkable global political commitment to combat the HIV/AIDS epidemic rapidly emerged at the United Nations.

HIV/AIDS featured prominently in the millennium development goals (MDGs) that emerged after the 2000 UN Millennium Summit and the Millennium Declaration which committed world leaders to combat poverty, hunger, disease, illiteracy, environmental degradation, and discrimination against women. Eight international development goals were set, with 21 targets to track progress. All 191 UN member states and at least 22 international organisations committed to help achieve the MDGs by 2015 (United Nations (UN), 2000a).

MDG 6 – to combat HIV/AIDS, malaria and other diseases – had two specific HIV/AIDS targets: 6A have halted by 2015 and begun to reverse the spread of HIV/AIDS; and 6B to achieve by 2010 universal access to treatment for HIV/AIDS for all those who need it. No other disease or health issue featured so prominently in the MDGs, nor had such specific targets and process indicators. In 2000, the Security Council (SC) also declared HIV/AIDS a security issue, underscoring that the pandemic, if unchecked, posed a risk to stability and security; and was exacerbated by conditions of violence and instability (United Nations (UN), 2000b). Global AIDS exceptionalism had truly arrived.

From 25 June to 27 June 2001, the 26th Special Session of the General Assembly of the United Nations (UNGASS) convened to discuss HIV/AIDS as a public health issue. The outcome document, the Declaration of Commitment on HIV/AIDS was negotiated by the governments of the world and served as a broad framework to guide national and international responses to address the global crisis as a matter of urgency (United Nations (UN), 2001).

Targets were set in key domains for action: political leadership; prevention, specified as the mainstay of the response; care, support and treatment, recognised as fundamental elements of an effective response; human rights; reducing vulnerability, particularly by empowering women; children orphaned and made vulnerable by the virus; alleviating social and economic impact; research and development, crucial with no vaccine or cure on the horizon; and addressing HIV/AIDS in conflict and disaster-effected regions.

The UNGASS Declaration was far-reaching in recognising that access to antiretroviral medicines was a fundamental element of the right of all people to the enjoyment of the highest attainable standard of health. It was specific that addressing the HIV/AIDS challenge could not be met without new, additional and sustained resources; that regular follow-up and reporting against specified targets were essential to maintain momentum and monitor progress. All this was predicated on a pivot towards a rights-based approach to global health (Gruskin & Tarantola, 2001).

Much quickly followed on, particularly in resource mobilisation. Having initially called for the creation of a Global Fund to fight AIDS at an African summit meeting in Abuja in April 2001, the G8 formally endorsed the proposal in July 2001 at its summit in Genoa in July 2001. The Global Fund, an international financing partnership to attract, leverage and invest additional resources to end the HIV/AIDS epidemic (subsequently broadened out to include tuberculosis (TB) and malaria) was established and began operations in January 2002 (Feachem & Sabot, 2006). The President's Emergency Plan for AIDS Relief (PEPFAR), a bilateral initiative of the US government, was launched by President George W. Bush in 2003. Since its inception, this has grown to become the largest global health program focused on a single disease in history, at least before the SARS-CoV-2/COVID 19 pandemic (Goosby et al., 2012).

Following UNGASS and reflecting on the commitments set out in the Millennium Declaration and crystallised into the MDGs, WHO held a series of consultative meetings. In June 2002 it published the first guidelines for scaling up ART in resource-limited settings (World Health Organization (WHO), 2002b). In late 2002, Dr Jong-wook Lee, WHO Director General, stated that lack of access to treatment was a global health emergency. He noted that to deliver ART to the millions who need it, we must change the way we think and the way we act, heralding the need for a radical new conceptualisation of public health action on HIV/AIDS. He believed in target-driven public health and advocated forcefully for ambitious treatment targets.

At the first UNGASS follow-up meeting, the UN General Assembly High-Level Meeting on HIV/AIDS in September 2003, WHO formally declared that the lack of access to HIV treatment was a global health emergency so as to stimulate action around the DOHA Declaration and promote access to affordable medicines for all (Lee, 2003). Antiretrovirals were increasingly positioned as essential medicines, but all had recently been developed and were under patent with strong price protection. Despite ARVs being regarded as essential medicines, maintaining the high prices set by originator companies rendered them unaffordable to the public sector in low- and middle-income countries (LMIC): one year of combination ART cost at least US$15,000 per patient in drug costs alone.

The DOHA Declaration, issued in November 2001, indicated that the Agreement on Trade-Related Aspects of Intellectual Property Rights (TRIPS), the international legal agreements between member nations of the World Trade Organization that governs intellectual property law should not prevent states from dealing with public health emergencies and allowed for compulsory licences to be issued (World Health Organization (WHO), 2002a). Declaring AIDS a public health crisis permitted flexibility in TRIPS. In particular, it stimulated several countries with local pharmaceutical manufacturing capacity to issue compulsory licences. Pharmaceutical companies in various developing countries were able to start production of lower-cost generic, as opposed to originator, antiretroviral medicines. Together with tiered pricing, where originator pharmaceutical companies offered lower price brand medicines to low- and low-middle income countries, annual treatment costs for combination ART started significantly to fall (World Health Organization (WHO), 2014a).

Conceptualising a new public health approach to HIV/AIDS care and treatment in the global south

Early treatment regimens were costly and cumbersome to take, with significant toxicity and tolerability issues for many patients. Single-agent therapy rapidly led to resistant virus and blunted efficacy. However, combining drugs together avoided the problem of drug resistance and when more potent drug classes became available in the mid-1990s, highly active combination ART was able effectively to suppress viral replication and retard disease progression, thus preventing the development of AIDS. The lived experience of people living with HIV was transformed from a death sentence to a long-term chronic disease.

Combination ART was complex and costly to deliver. Patients were individually managed by expert specialist AIDS physicians often based in tertiary-level hospitals where they were backed up by state-of-the-art high-technology laboratory and diagnostic services. Access to such effective therapy was largely restricted to high-income countries with sophisticated health services that could afford the high costs of treatment, provide the necessary laboratory support for monitoring, and had sufficient capacity, particularly human resources for health to effectively deploy ART.

In stark contrast in low-income settings, particularly sub-Saharan Africa which was bearing the brunt of the pandemic, very few health services had the capacity or resources to provide such expensive specialised care and treatment in the public sector. Access to effective ART or specific OI disease prophylaxis was very limited; where available it was largely restricted to urban elites accessing individualised private healthcare in third-level hospitals.

Often unrecognised or undiagnosed, HIV disease and AIDS continued to rampage through urban and rural communities, overwhelming public-sector hospitals and healthcare services. The spectrum of HIV-related diseases was very different: chronic diarrhoea and wasting (slim disease), TB and non-opportunistic bacterial infections predominated. Patients were dying much earlier on in the clinical course of their HIV infection, with high-grade pathogens, limited treatment and care and overwhelmed health services (C. F. Gilks, 1993). Health inequity had rarely been more obvious.

At the global level, there was growing concern about the widening disparities in HIV disease rates and AIDS survival between the global north, where the epidemic was concentrated in high-risk communities; and the global south, where infection was more prevalent and generalised. And an emerging consensus that something had to be done, and quickly, to address this profound health inequity. As this pivot towards a global exceptional AIDS response gained momentum, it became obvious that existing, limited health systems in the global south could not take on the existing burden of HIV/AIDS and deliver effective individualised care and treatment to all in need.

Radical thinking to conceptualise a new public health approach to HIV/AIDS was therefore necessary if ART was ever to be widely accessible to all in need through the public health sector:

- This would require a significant pivot in the global health architecture from traditional public health action, typically concerned with communicable and other disease prevention and control at the population level through primary healthcare (PHC) to include hospital facilities providing specialist clinical services and all cadres of health professionals.
- Patient care and ART was regarded as highly specialised in the global north. To address inequity, the focus had to shift to a simplified and standardised population-level approach, accessible to those in need from an individualised case management approach led by specialist physicians and accessible only to a minority. It needed to be across the life-course.
- If ART were ever to be rolled out, it would have to be initiated in district hospitals or tertiary facilities and could only link with PHC delivery points when the patient's disease was stabilised, and ART was tolerated. Most ARVs would be dispensed from hospital-based pharmacies. In the traditional

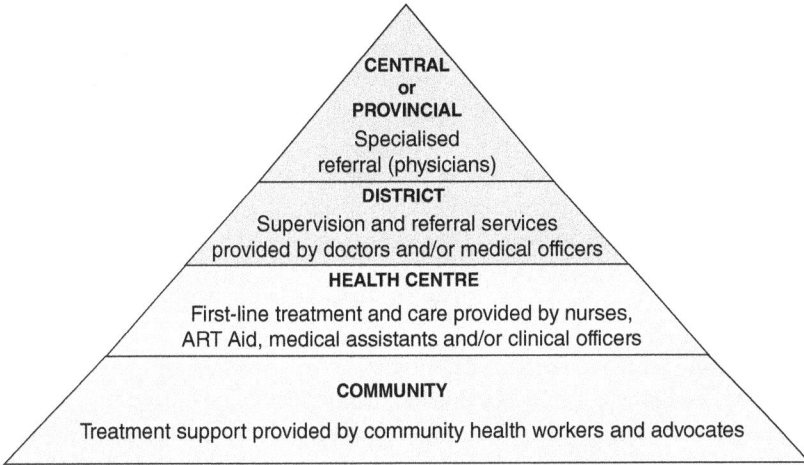

Figure 1.1 The traditional hierarchy of care for ART delivery

pyramidal hierarchy of healthcare delivery, the key focus for population-wide ART would need to move from the apex to the lower levels of service delivery and community, where most care and treatment would be delivered.
• Guideline development would require blurring of the traditional boundaries between public health and clinical medicine, needing inputs from specialist physicians who understood ART and hospital-based care integrated with inputs from public health practitioners who understood PHC through four delivery platforms: community health workers; health centres, first-level hospitals, mobile services.
• Huge investments would be required in human resources for health and for purchasing HIV diagnostics, appropriate technology and antiretroviral and other medicines. To make treatment widely accessible, ART and AIDS care would need to be decentralised out to communities and delivered by primary care services. Given the complexities of AIDS care and treatment and specialist care services, these investments had first to be made at the secondary care level and then widen out to the primary care level. Hospital pharmacies and laboratory facilities were often in need of significant rehabilitation. Inevitably health system strengthening had to involve hospitals and not start and remain at the primary care level (Figure 1.1).

Towards universal access to antiretroviral therapy (ART)

In late 2003, WHO with UNAIDS launched the global Initiative to provide ART to 3 million people with HIV/AIDS in developing countries by the end of 2005, thereby setting the first global targets to expand treatment (World Health

Organization (WHO), 2003b). Many were surprised by this bold leadership around "3by5", as it came to be known, and were unconvinced that the WHO strategy to make it happen was either feasible or achievable. It did however mark a sea change in global HIV/AIDS policy, ensuring that AIDS treatment was now seen as equally important as HIV prevention.

The "3by5" initiative was a clear affirmation that the right to health also included access to healthcare, something people living with HIV across the globe understood and welcomed. There was very limited community support for a prevention only approach, excluding those infected, sick and dying from any specific HIV/AIDS interventions. It would take a while to convince sceptics that we couldn't treat our way out of the epidemic; or that we couldn't afford even to try. It also worried some public health practitioners who were concerned that the global health agenda had become too medicalised (Clark, 2014) – though it is hard to see how scaling up ART could be achieved without the application of an overt biomedical process involving reductionism, individualism and a focus on medical treatment and outcome.

In July 2005, the G8 held its 31st summit at Gleneagles, Scotland. At the forum, leaders from Canada, the European Commission, France, Germany, Italy, Japan, Russia, the United Kingdom and the United States (the richest Industrialised nations in the global north) came together with leaders from the global south. The summit was considered one of the most productive held. In the communique, paragraph 18(d) is noteworthy: "with the aim of an AIDS-free generation in Africa, significantly reducing HIV infections and working with WHO, UNAIDS and other international bodies to develop and implement a package for HIV prevention, treatment and care, with the aim of as close as possible to universal access to treatment for all those who need it by 2010" (G8 Gleneagles, 2005).

This exceptional global commitment to universal access in the fight against HIV/AIDS was taken up by the UN General Assembly in June 2006, following the High-level review on AIDS. The resolution adopted by the General Assembly, the Political Declaration on HIV/AIDS, represented a consensus of Heads of State and Government and leaders from all parts of the world to pursue all necessary efforts to scale up national responses in order to achieve universal access to comprehensive prevention programmes, treatment care and support by 2010 (United Nations (UN), 2006). Several UN high-level meetings followed, aiming to keep countries on track to achieve universal access.

Nested in these unprecedented developments in the global health architecture at the start of the millennium was a deep commitment to social justice and the right to health, defined broadly in the 1946 Constitution of WHO as "the enjoyment of the highest attainable standard of health", with a growing focus on the right to healthcare. It was a new embodiment of PHC, and the need to make this universal and accessible to all individuals and families in a community, with a strong focus on health equity (Van Lerberghe, 2008). It was also a significant evolution in the way health systems were operating, as universal access to ART would need to encompass secondary specialist services fully integrated with primary care.

Drivers of the response for global AIDS exceptionalism

To date, five health-related topics have now been discussed at UN General Assembly Special Sessions and subsequent high-level meetings: the first was HIV/AIDS in 2001; then non-communicable diseases (NCDs) in 2011; antimicrobial resistance (AMR) in 2016; tuberculosis (TB) in 2018; and universal health coverage (UHC) in 2019. Interestingly, the success of the increased international commitment that was evident after the HIV/AIDS UNGASS meeting in 2001 was also seen, albeit to a much lesser degree, with NCDs and AMR, but have not significantly been realised for either TB or UHC (Rodi et al., 2022). Aside from PEPFAR and the Global Fund, no new funding mechanisms nor significant additional resource allocations have emerged. Nor has anything akin to the UN Political Declaration on HIV/AIDS emerged for these other health issues.

The global alliance for vaccines and immunisation (GAVI), now Gavi, the Vaccine Alliance, is the only other significant global health initiative (GHI) and public-private partnership to match PEPFAR or the Global Fund. It grew from the Children's Vaccine Initiative (CVI), launched in 1990 after the World Summit for Children with a specific remit to accelerate efforts to develop vaccines that could enhance the performance of the expanded programme on immunisation (EPI), now housed in WHO (Mitchell et al., 1993).

Of note, the SARS-CoV-2/Covid-19 pandemic has yet to figure meaningfully at the UN (Farrall & Michaelsen, 2021). Swiftly declared by WHO as a public health emergency of international concern (PHEIC), member states responded rapidly to curtail travel, introduce lockdowns and other public health interventions to reduce transmission; and develop effective treatments and preventive vaccines at the national level. Under the 2005 International Health Regulations (IHR), countries are required to notify WHO of an extraordinary event that may have a significant risk of international spread; WHO then formally declares a PHEIC. There have been to date seven declarations: 2009 H1N1 swine flu pandemic; 2014 polio; 2013–2016 West Africa Ebola outbreak; 2015–2016 Zika epidemic; 2018-2-20 Kivu Ebola epidemic; the ongoing COVID-19 pandemic; and the 2022–2023 Mpox (formerly Monkeypox) outbreak (Merianos & Peiris, 2005). Interestingly HIV/AIDS has never been regarded as a PHEIC, nor was it considered a notifiable disease under the previous 1969 IHRs.

Given this, it is important to ask why HIV/AIDS has been so frequently been discussed at the UN and so conspicuously successful in spawning GHIs without being declared a PHEIC by WHO to understand and identify the drivers of global AIDS exceptionalism; and to draw lessons for NCDs and UHC, as we do in Sections 2 and 3. How and why did this come about; what needs to be done by other disease control programmes and emerging global health priorities to step up commitments and resourcing to deliver results that can impact communities and individuals? (Table 1.1).

The main drivers of the HIV response have undoubtedly come from the community and the new forms of disease advocacy and activism they developed. Outspoken civil society activists and patient-led organisations embodied GIPA and were very vocal in their demands: something needed to be done and urgently to change the status quo so as more effectively to combat the epidemic that was killing so many friends and partners; and scaring the general public. Community support groups sprang up to provide care and support to individuals isolated and excluded because of overt stigma and discrimination and to households impoverished by AIDS.

They aligned closely with alarmed public health officials and agencies to call for robust responses to confront the prejudice, stigma and discrimination that were significant impediments and obstacles to action. They provided appropriate care and support interventions; and aggressively advocated for fast-track research and development into AIDS treatments and HIV vaccines. Enlightened politicians, starting in the United Sates listened to these passionate and often angry voices.

The United Nations led by alarmed member states responded, discussed HIV/AIDS, recognised the inequity in response and considered what to do. Concerted action followed: an exceptional response above and beyond normal health interventions rapidly emerged to protect the rights of those at special risk, to generate resources to assist and support affected communities and sufficient to start to control the HIV epidemic.

The first organisation was the Gay Men's Health Crisis (GMHC), a New York City-based community-based AIDS service organisation founded in January 1982: its mission is to end the AIDS epidemic and uplift the lives of all affected. Crisis counselling, legal aid, volunteer supporters and the buddy system were some of the innovations GMHC pioneered (Kayal, 2018). One of the best known and most activist pressure groups was ACT UP – the AIDS Coalition to Unleash Power. It was founded in New York in 1987 and has become an international grassroots political group working towards the end of AIDS. The early years of its activities are well discussed in a prize-winning book by Sarah Schulman "Let the record show: a political history of ACT UP New York 1987–1993" (Schulman, 2021). Several other influential groups have emerged in the United States with differing agendas. Most notably is the treatment action group (TAG), an independent, activist community-based research and policy think tank. It initially focussed on fighting to end HIV, but now includes TB and hepatitis C virus (HCV) (Chou et al., 2009).

This energy and activism also took hold in the global south, particularly in countries where HIV/AIDS was rampant. The AIDS Support Organisation

Table 1.1 Key meetings on HIV and AIDS at the UN, WHO, UNAIDS and G8

Year	UN, G8, WHO or UNAIDS meeting	Outcome
1987	AIDS becomes the first disease ever debated at the UN General Assembly	The UN registers deep concern about AIDS and commends WHO's leadership and efforts towards global AIDS prevention and control
2000	4172nd meeting of the UN Security Council	The HIV/AIDS pandemic, if unchecked, declared a risk to peace and security in Africa
2000	The UN Millennium Summit	The Millenium Declaration with MDG 6 to combat HIV/AIDS, malaria and other diseases
2001	26th Special Session of the General Assembly of the UN (UNGASS)	Declaration of Commitment on HIV/AIDS Support for a Global HIV/AIDS Health Fund
2001	G8 Summit at Genoa, Italy	The Global Fund established to invest new resources to end the HIV/AIDS epidemic
2003	First UN General Assembly High-Level Meeting on HIV/AIDS	Lack of access to ART is declared a global health emergency
2003	WHO & UNAIDS strategy meeting to provide ART to developing countries	The "3by5" initiative launched
2005	G8 Summit at Gleneagles, Scotland	Universal access to ART for all those who need it by 2010
2006	UN General Assembly High-Level Meeting on HIV/AIDS	Political Declaration towards universal access to HIV prevention, treatment, care, support
2011	UN General Assembly High-Level Meeting on HIV/AIDS	Political Declaration on HIV/AIDS intensifying efforts to eliminate HIV/AIDS; UNAIDS getting to zero strategy: zero discrimination; new infections; AIDS deaths
2014	UNAIDS calls for ambitious treatment target to help end the AIDS epidemic	UNAIDS treatment targets for 2020: 90% with HIV are diagnosed; 90% diagnosed on ART; 90% on ART with suppressed viral loads
2015	UN General Assembly meeting on the 2030 sustainable development agenda	Creation of the 17 Sustainable Development Goals and the 2030 agenda for sustainable development

(Continued)

Table 1.1 (Continued)

Year	UN, G8, WHO or UNAIDS meeting	Outcome
2015	UNAIDS accelerating fast-track action to end the AIDS epidemic by 2030	New UNAIDS fast-track 95/95/95 targets for diagnosis, treatment and viral suppression
2016	UN General Assembly High-Level Meeting on HIV/AIDS	UN Political Declaration on HIV/AIDS on the Fast-Track to accelerate the fight against HIV and end the AIDS epidemic by 2030
2021	2021 UN General Assembly High-Level Meeting on AIDS	UN Political Declaration on HIV/AIDS ending inequalities, getting on track to end AIDS by 2030

(TASO), founded in Uganda in 1987, was one of the first community support organisations in Africa and is probably the most influential. The story of how it started is illustrative and well-articulated by the founder Noerine Kaleeba in her 1991 book "We miss you all. Noerine Kaleeba: AIDS in the family". Now out of print, insights and excerpts are available in an informative book review in Reproductive Health Matters (Kaleeba & Ray, 2003).

Close behind, the Treatment Action Campaign was founded in South Africa by a well-known PLHA and community activist Zachie Achmat. Leading with courage and by example, he steadfastly refused to start ART until 2003 when it was being made widely available according to need across South Africa. Its vision is a unified health system that provides equal access to quality and dignified healthcare services for all including people who are living with HIV and TB (Szijarto, 2023).

Non-governmental organisations (NGOs) have long been central to Brazil's strong response to HIV/AIDS. One of the oldest and most prominent is the Brazilian Interdisciplinary AIDS Association or ABIA, which was founded in 1987 (Cueto & Lopes, 2023). Organisations with shared objectives and visions around HIV/AIDS have also started to come together. The best known is ICASO – the International Council of AIDS Service Organisations which was founded in 1991. Based in Canada its vision is an end to the HIV epidemic for all. Its mission statement is to mobilise communities to provide transformative leadership in response to HIV and intersecting challenges. Civil society organisations have a prominent role in GHIs, are increasingly consulted by international organisations and can act as conduits for funding (Doyle & Patel, 2008).

More recently in the global south, civil society has started to focus on key and priority populations particularly MSM and transgender communities. A good example of this is APCOM: founded in 2006 and based in Bangkok, it is a not-for-profit organisation representing and working with a network of individuals and community-based organisations across 35 countries in the Asia Pacific region. The primary focus is on HIV as a key health issue for gay men and MSM, but it also addresses sexual and mental health and drug use (Garcia & Koerner, 2014).

So, the scene was set for action. Civil society's voice that ART must be widely accessible for all according to need rather than affordability or the ability to pay had been listened to. The political will was there, funds were available, The UN, G8 WHO had set the goal of universal access to ART. HIV/AIDS policy was rapidly evolving and expectations were high: health and healthcare for all. The public health sector in the global south was primed. But it was unclear what was to be done and quite how this could practically be achieved.

2 "3by5" – coming to grips with the AIDS treatment gap

The multiple challenges facing global ART scale-up

When the UN Millennium Declaration in 2000 committed member states to combat poverty, hunger, disease, illiteracy, environmental degradation and discrimination against women, it was clear that health was central in what was a mutually reinforcing framework for human development (United Nations (UN), 2000a). This was particularly the case with poverty reduction because of the well-documented impact of ill-health on poverty through loss of income, catastrophic health expenditure and orphanhood. At the same time, the WHO Commission on Macroeconomics and Health showed that good health is essential to sustainable development (Waitzkin, 2003). With three of the eight millennium development goals (MDGs) health-related, no-one could claim that development was just about economic growth.

Sceptics questioned the value of the ambitious MDG health goals, particularly the specific HIV/AIDS prevention and treatment targets: 6A, to have halted by 2015 and begun to reverse the spread of HIV/AIDS; 6B, to achieve by 2010 universal access to treatment for HIV/AIDS for all those who need it. There was further concern that an intense new focus on hospital-based services to deliver on the treatment target would detract from HIV prevention, the previous sole priority for AIDS control, and inhibit progress towards halting and beginning to reverse the spread of HIV/AIDS by 2015.

Shortages of health services and other public sector staff was a critical challenge, and it was clear that any improvement in health outcomes in general, and HIV/AIDS in particular, depended on major improvements in healthcare delivery systems (Haines & Cassels, 2004). Regardless of whether staff were deployed for HIV prevention or to provide ART (rarely initially for both) there were insufficient health professionals to impact the pandemic. Despite huge support for global AIDS exceptionalism, most outside WHO felt these were laudatory aspirational goals with little chance of success.

Few had confidence that the essential pivot to making ART universally accessible to all in need was feasible in high HIV-burden countries in the global

DOI: 10.4324/9781003505693-4

south: with limited capacity, few countries could effectively translate aspirational policy goals into practical outcomes. Even with Global Fund and PEPFAR resources, providing ART would be very complex, costly and challenging to deliver. With the public sector as both the purchaser of ARVs and diagnostics and the sole provider of treatment, there were few opportunities for incentives to lead to cost containment, organisational flexibility, greater efficiency and improved service quality (Tynkkynen et al., 2013).

Health services across Africa were being overwhelmed by the sheer volume of sick, young AIDS patients while the existing burden of disease was in no way diminishing (Gilks et al., 1998). Patients were dying, health staff had little specific to offer except palliation, and morale was crashing; burn-out was common and staff were leaving in droves. Workers who remained in post were themselves falling sick with HIV/AIDS: facilities were experiencing grave staffing problems with chronic ill-health and time off work compounded by posts being blocked, and high staff death rates. These additional pressures on the public health sector further compromised performance and service delivery.

Most donors and funding agencies were concentrating on HIV prevention at the community and primary care level. Clearly HIV care and treatment could not just be practiced at this level; indeed ART was, at least at the start of scale-up, almost entirely hospital-based with a strong focus on individual case management. Most public health practitioners were familiar with primary healthcare delivering preventative services and a relatively simple package of primary care interventions across communities and populations. Few had practical clinical experience or familiarity with specialist treatment and patient care at the secondary or tertiary level. Nor did they interact closely or work with hospital-based clinicians and specialists.

Integrating these two groups with different cultures and approaches to health and disease was a significant challenge but was critical: public health ART needed better integration of primary care and second-level hospital care for it to be effectively delivered for the long-term, lifelong and across the life course. Commentators have noted that the response to the pandemic eventually disrupted the traditional boundaries between public health and clinical medicine (Brandt, 2013).

There was a further challenge with the cadre of specialist AIDS physicians largely from the global north who were providing expert advice on ART to National Health Authorities, bilateral bodies like PEPFAR and multilateral agencies, particularly WHO. Their expertise was gained in well-resourced settings, focused on individual case management and was supported by sophisticated laboratory services. The guidelines they were familiar with and had provided input into were masterful and comprehensive but were more akin to specialist physician manuals for practitioners in well-resourced settings than practical guidelines for healthcare workers to use in low-income settings.

Few were familiar with the capacity constraints facing health services in the global south as they started ART scale-up with severe limitations in financing, drug management systems, appropriately trained healthcare personnel, facilities and laboratory services. Often with little background in public health, moving away from the individual patient to a population-level approach was a significant conceptual shift: relatively few were comfortable with this change in perspective, failing to recognise that scaling up ART in the global south was impossible without this paradigm shift.

The final challenge was the enormity of the task in hand. The resource needs for effective HIV/AIDS prevention and care needs were far below what was available in low- and middle-income countries (Schwartländer et al., 2001). In 2003, WHO estimated that just under 6 million adults in developing countries were in need of immediate treatment but that only about 400,000 were on treatment, with the majority from just one country Brazil. While Africa was bearing the brunt of the AIDS epidemic, ART coverage was at best 2% (World Health Organization (WHO), 2003b).

There were relatively few healthcare professionals, and most were based in large towns and cities: almost none working in the public sector had received training in ART and AIDS clinical management. Massive investments needed rapidly to be made in human resources for health and to strengthen weak and overstretched health system capacity, far in excess of the limited initial funds coming from the Global Fund and PEPFAR. The absorptive capacity for major resource inputs into health was expected to be a significant rate-limiting step in many settings.

Making a start with the WHO "3by5" initiative

Despite widespread scepticism and the multiple challenges involved in delivering ART to all in need in the global south, a start had to be made. As the technical agency in the UN tasked with health, WHO felt it incumbent upon itself to take the lead. In 2003, under the newly appointed Director General Dr Lee Jong-wook, WHO began work with UNAIDS on the "3by5" strategy, a global initiative to provide ART to 3 million people with HIV/AIDS in developing countries by the end of 2005. Dr Lee had already stated that global efforts to control HIV/AIDS would be the right course to give meaning to his tenure as WHO DG. Dr Lee died prematurely in 2006. It is important that we recognise and remember his leadership role in the "3by5" Initiative and acknowledge it as his signature strategy.

The "3by5" initiative was outlined in a game-changing publication "Treating 3 million by 2005; Making it happen; the WHO strategy". In the introduction, Dr Peter Piot, Executive Director of UNAIDS, noted "the formidable barrier of creating sufficient operational capacity" to expand access to HIV treatment; and that the target was "a massive challenge but one we cannot afford to miss."

Dr Lee noted that "lack of access to antiretroviral treatment is a global health emergency... To deliver antiretroviral treatment to the millions who need it, we must change the way we think and change the way we act." For those involved then it was clear that this was an organisation-wide priority and was critically not UN business as usual (World Health Organization (WHO), 2003b).

Because "3by5" set the scene for everything that followed, it is worth reviewing the elements that were outlined in what became a major, influential policy document. It embodied several guiding principles: urgency; equity; the centrality of people living with HIV/AIDS; the provision of lifelong care; treatment and human rights; accountability; country ownership; sustainability; and partnership and plurality. In retrospect, these now seem obvious; at the time they were radical and exceptional.

As a roadmap to improve ART access and scale-up delivery, it had an aspirational and unambiguous goal; and a single, clear, highly ambitious, time-bound target. Both were unequivocally welcomed by activists and infected and affected communities in the global north and south.

The goal of the Initiative is for WHO and its partners to make the greatest possible contribution to prolonging the survival and restoring the quality of life of individuals with HIV/AIDS, advancing to the ultimate goal of universal access to ART for those in need of care, as a human right and within the context of a comprehensive response to HIV/AIDS.

The target of the Initiative is by the end of 2005, 3 million eligible people in developing countries who need ART will be receiving effective antiretroviral therapy.

The five pillars of the "3by5" strategic framework

Recognising that delivering "3by5" would require concerted and accelerated action by many actors, WHO in consultation with partners and key stakeholders developed a strategic framework with five pillars and 14 key strategic elements. Scaling up ART from a very low base was a multidimensional challenge, therefore the framework was relatively complex. WHO drew on the successful expansion of TB control and the roll-out of the Integrated Management of Childhood Illness (IMCI) programme to note that seemingly daunting challenges could be met (World Health Organization (WHO), 2004a).

The five pillars represent the thinking behind the Initiative; how it would be operationalised; and the tactics WHO and partners would need to adopt to overcome the numerous challenges to meet the aspirational goal and ambitious treatment target:

Pillar one: global leadership, alliances and advocacy. The most vital work will happen in countries and communities; global alliances and advocacy will be crucial enablers. UNAIDS has driven and catalysed growing international determination to respond to the HIV/AIDS crisis, including the area of treatment access. Working with UNAIDS and alongside other partners, WHO will step forward and fully exercise its specific responsibility for the health sector – above all in advocating treatment.

Pillar two: urgent, sustained country support. The success of ART programmes depends on scaled up country action. Countries must drive the process of expanding HIV/AIDS treatment: their specific needs and capacities will shape strategy and determine activities. WHO will provide implementers with essential technical and policy advice and tools and will cooperate with countries at every stage in designing and implementing national plans for scaling up ART.

Pillar three: simplified, standardised tools for delivering ART. Rapidly scaling up ART requires user-friendly guidelines to help health workers identify and enrol people living with HIV/AIDS, deliver therapy and monitor results. Providing these guidelines and updating them as new information comes in is a central part of WHO's role.

Pillar four: effective, reliable supply of medicines and diagnostics. The viability of ART programmes depends on a reliable, efficiently managed supply of quality medicines and diagnostics procured at a sustainable cost. WHO recognises the importance of drug procurement and supply management for scaling up ART and the challenges many countries and providers face. A key action is to establish an AIDS Medicines and Diagnostics Service (AMDS).

Pillar five: rapidly identifying and reapplying new knowledge and success. Successful organisations apply experimentation, innovation and real-time learning with rapid diffusion. The many challenges with ART scale-up requires a robust programme to consistently learn, document, share and act.

The 14 strategic elements in the five pillars are noted in Table 2.1. Along with clear goals, targets and guiding principles, they have contemporary relevance to policymakers moving priority agendas forward; to national planners and policymakers implementing vertical disease control programmes; and to global health students seeking to understand how agendas are built and realised.

Turning strategic thinking into programmatic action and realisable outcomes

Each pillar had key WHO actions: some were context-specific, others are now standard practice. Most were successfully enacted to turn strategic thinking into practical activities and realisable outcomes, many of which are still programmatically relevant. It may be WHO-centric to focus on these, but the "3by5" Initiative was a transformative policy document with goals, targets and guiding principles; and WHO was holding itself accountable for delivery. This was beyond the normative and technical work WHO traditionally did; it was however reliant on its convening role to bring partners and stakeholders to the table and align them to common purpose within the "3by5" Initiative.

Table 2.1 The "3by5" five strategic pillars and strategic elements

"3by5" strategic pillar	"3by5" strategic element
Pillar one: Global leadership, strong partnership and advocacy	1. Visible WHO leadership and commitment to urgent action to reach the goal of universal access to ART 2. Locate the "3by5" Initiative within the broader development context 3. Support all countries in scaling up ART, while focusing WHO efforts on the high-burden countries in greatest need 4. Align and mobilise partner support and the private sector to achieve the "3by5" target at the global level
Pillar two: Urgent, sustained country support	5. Secure the key elements required at the national level to deliver the "3by5" target as part of a comprehensive response to HIV/AIDS and accelerate prevention 6. Strengthen and support the renewal of health systems and national operational capacity for scaling up ART 7. Strengthen and build human capacity for scaling up ART 8. Strengthen the capacity of affected communities, including vulnerable groups living with HIV/AIDS, to be fully involved in planning and delivering ART programmes
Pillar three: Simplified and standardised tools for ART delivery	9. Simplify and standardise procedures to identify individuals who need therapy and to facilitate entry into ART programmes 10. Simplify and standardise ART to facilitate adherence and to enable rapid scaling up to be implemented 11. Simplify and standardise tools for tracking the performance of ART programmes including surveillance of drug resistance
Pillar four: Reliable supply of medicines and diagnostics	12. Support country access to and the reliable, efficient distribution of high-quality low-cost medicines and diagnostics
Pillar five: Rapidly identifying and reapplying new knowledge and success	13. Build on success 14. Continuously learn by doing – with ongoing evaluation and analysis of programme performance and a focus on operational research

Undoubtedly in Pillar one, WHO's highly visible leadership was key in spurring urgent action towards universal access to ART; and getting all partners and stakeholders in health aligned around their specific roles in "3by5". ART scale-up was conclusively located within the broader development context. With UNAIDS, ethical guidelines were published promoting equity in ART (Joint United Nations Programme on HIV/AIDS (UNAIDS), 2006). Work to close the global funding gap was started and still continues today, albeit with many more partners and agencies actively involved. WHO's technical leadership in HIV/AIDS remains critically important today.

With WHO's constitution and governance structure (the primacy of the World Health Assembly and each member state Minister of Health's voice and vote) it was clear for Pillar two that the Initiative would develop and sustain strong country support. The speed with which a common commitment to "3by5" targets and processes from all participating countries was secured was unprecedented. This led to the rapid deployment of WHO teams with appropriate technical skills and knowledge to each country, training health and community workers in ART delivery and strengthening laboratories in collaboration with partners and funders. Although the days of the "3by5" missions are long gone, the need for ongoing training and strengthening laboratory and hospital infrastructure and capacity remains; the work started in "3by5" continues.

The deliverables under Pillar three were all achieved. Multiple entry points identified PLHA in need of treatment and a start was made in the development of simple standard testing procedures, technical guidelines, methods to track drug resistance and monitor and evaluate ART delivery systems: all continue today within WHO and partners. The public health approach emerged from the guideline process, and has been reviewed by WHO to consider how to adapt it to current challenges and opportunities (Ford et al., 2018).

The deliverables under Pillar four all relate to procurement and supply of high-quality low-cost ARVs and diagnostics. WHO established an AMDS providing demand forecasts and information on legal issues, prices, and sources; and supported countries in forecasting, procurement, management and distribution. Given its centrality to ART scale-up, other partners, agencies and implementers (notably PEPFAR in PEPFAR countries) now provide support for procurement and distribution of medicines and diagnostics at country and global levels. WHO has concentrated on prequalification working in close collaboration with national regulatory agencies and other partner organisations to make quality priority medical products available for those who urgently need them. Its remit now includes malaria, TB, reproductive health, hepatitis, diarrhoeal diseases and selected neglected tropical diseases (NTDs) as well as HIV/AIDS (World Health Organization (WHO), 2019).

The deliverables under Pillar five, learning by doing and new knowledge generation then rapidly getting new research into policy and practice remain fundamental to ART scale up and indeed to any disease control programme. While

WHO remains a stakeholder and committed to learning by doing, there has been an explosion of operational research largely supported by research bodies in the global north with the funds and capacity to fund and conduct the research. WHO retains a key role in convening guideline development expert panels and technical groups to review new evidence; and documenting and disseminating successful models from country experiences.

"3by5": a bold start or an inevitable failure?

As the "3by5" initiative started, the 2004 World Health Report, boldly entitled "Changing History", was published. WHO DG Dr Lee was clear that future generations will judge our era in large part by our response to the AIDS pandemic. There were unprecedented opportunities for health with important technological advances and the flow of international investment in health, most of which was for HIV/AIDS, greatly improving the prospects for pandemic control. The responsibility of WHO and partners was to ensure that the increased funding enabled countries to fight HIV/AIDS while simultaneously strengthening their health systems: "3by5" would accelerate this process. WHO was fully aware that the stakes were high and that it was taking significant risks embracing a time-limited difficult goal that would change the way WHO worked. There was huge optimism that "3by5" could work (World Health Organization (WHO), 2004b).

From the start, "3by5" had its detractors. The global resource needs for HIV/AIDS prevention and care estimated that six million PLHA were in immediate need of ART (Schwartländer et al., 2001). The three million target was based on an ambitious assessment that half could access treatment by the end of 2005; and was regarded by WHO and UNAIDS as a necessary, achievable target towards the ultimate goal of universal access to ART. Some saw the target as totally unrealistic, and that it was far too ambitious. Others worried that there had been no discussion about how the figure was derived and that it was not ambitious enough.

Whether "3by5" was the best approach to tackling the HIV pandemic was debated in the literature (Kim & Ammann, 2004). The critics accepted that improving access to life-saving ART was a moral imperative, but that there were three fundamental problems with the "3by5" approach: it had far too narrow a focus just on ART; costs would constantly escalate to sustain ART scale-up and delivery; it was top-down and by-passed country ownership and NGO engagement. AIDS exceptionalism was not warranted. WHO's view was that scaling up treatment was not only a possibility but a reality. The Initiative was a point of entry to combating the epidemic with four clear principles at its heart: treatment must be a core element; time is of the essence; clear consensus targets are indispensable; and guidance to combat HIV must be codified and simplified. WHO then posed the question – what would be the likely cost if it were never attempted?

As the Initiative progressed, disappointingly modest increases in the number of people on ART were recorded. It was proving difficult to keep down ARV prices; few African governments were using the flexibilities in international law to make essential medicines more affordable; generic manufacturers were not registering or manufacturing antiretrovirals; and there was little use of tiered pricing. By the end of 2005, only about 1.3 million people in low- and middle-income countries were receiving ART; nearly 5 million people became infected in 2005; and while perhaps 300,000 lives had been saved by ART, conservatively three million people globally still died with AIDS in 2005 (Bongaarts, 2006). The Lancet concluded that "3by5" will be remembered for its failure. But it did also note that the Initiative should also be applauded for its extraordinary political successes, particularly spurring world leaders to agree to the goal of universal access to treatment by 2010 (Lancet, 2005).

WHO and UNAIDS agreed, recognising in March 2006 that the target had not been met on time for a variety of reasons. The global public health paradigm does not easily change: social and economic conditions that have caused the collapse of public health systems cannot be corrected overnight; inadequate healthcare infrastructure and shortages of trained workers, affordable drugs and diagnostics will still hamper public health efforts for years to come; stigma and discrimination remain as two of the most stubborn obstacles. Nevertheless "3by5" confirmed that ART can be provided even in the most challenging settings; the number accessing ART is on an upward trajectory, most noticeable in sub-Saharan Africa. The global dialogue on access to treatment has changed for good and with this our hope of tackling not just HIV but other diseases of poverty as well (World Health Organization (WHO), 2006d) (Figure 2.1).

Unfortunately, just days after the untimely death of WHO DG Dr Lee, the pharmaceutical industry continued to criticise "3by5". The most noteworthy was an opinion piece in the New York Times written by Dr Carol Adelman from the Hudson Institute, Washington entitled "let's learn from global health failures" (Adelman, 2006). She opined that the greatest tribute to Dr Lee would be a new commitment to implementing policies that work. WHO had allowed advocacy to triumph science: focusing on patents and high originator drug prices as barriers to ART use, it recommended using copies of AIDS drugs produced by generic manufacturers with unknown safety and efficacy, and ignored the opportunities offered by tiered pricing. Without evidence, she claimed that substandard and counterfeit generics were contributing to the emergence of drug-resistant strains of HIV.

WHO commissioned an independent evaluation of its contribution to "3by5". The expert team noted that ART is not only a technical consideration: it must be seen in the context of global development processes such as poverty reduction, the 2001 UNGASS declaration and the MDGs. They recognised that important progress had been made although the numbers on ART was less than half the target; prevention efforts were not impacting transmission; and many of the

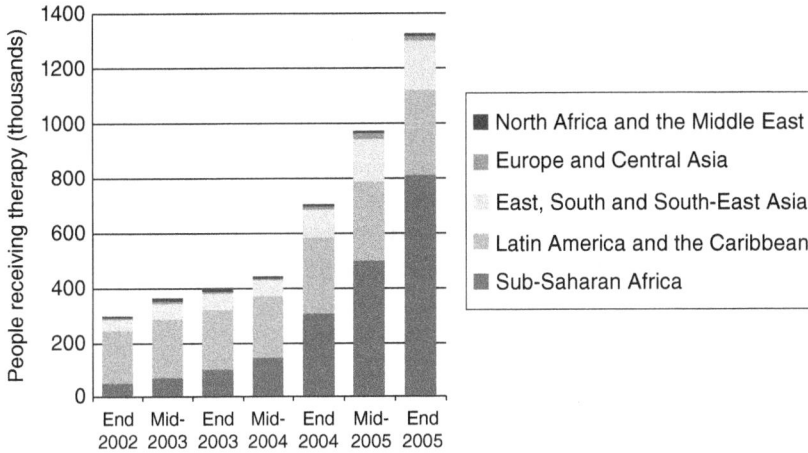

Source: WHO/UNAIDS (2006). Progress on global access to HIV antiretroviral therapy: An update on "3 by 5."

Figure 2.1 Numbers receiving ART by WHO region over the "3by5" period 2002–2005

worst-affected countries were far from containing their AIDS crises. It credited the Initiative with establishing ART as an essential public health intervention. A total of 38 specific recommendations across the five strategic pillars were made, all to strengthen WHO's position in the highly politicised environment of development cooperation and to ensure that the Universal Access goal does not follow "3by5" in missing the target (Battistella Nemes et al., 2006).

A much more recent reflection on "3by5" has concluded that it failed due to technical and political reasons. The commentators did not consider any impact beyond 2005. They noted the deadline was too short; it was an ineffective tool for achieving a balance between prevention and treatment or for strengthening national health systems. Politically, WHO had not done enough to address the level of denial and silence around AIDS nor to fight discrimination against PLHA and minority groups. And while there was a strong human-rights perspective in Geneva it did not clearly get translated into practical activities in a programme that was characterised as focussing on drug distribution. Operating in a complex and sometimes adverse political context it became overshadowed and dominated by PEPFAR (Cueto et al., 2019).

A fairer reflection would acknowledge that a bold start had been made to treatment scale-up that was aspirational and ambitious and likely to fail. A start had to be made: it was impossible for WHO not to respond and then be ill-judged by history for such a failure to act. The costs of inaction would have been catastrophic in terms of AIDS deaths and an uncontrolled pandemic. ART would not have been established as an essential public health intervention, nor would the unstoppable momentum for ART scale-up been realised. Years come and go; in fact, 3 million persons were receiving ART in low- and middle-income countries by the end of 2007 and a "3by7" Initiative would not have been a failure (Joint United Nations Programme on HIV/AIDS (UNAIDS), 2008).

Imitation is the sincerest form of flattery, and at the UN General Assembly, the 2011 update of the Political Declaration on HIV/AIDS to intensify efforts to eliminate HIV/AIDS included a new combined number/date target of "15by15" (United Nations (UN), 2011). This time the target was met nine months ahead of schedule, another clear but undisputed example of the merits and value of target-driven public health in HIV/AIDS programming (World Health Organization (WHO), 2015c).

3 Unpacking the WHO public health approach to ART

A pragmatic start: standardised regimens and simplified formularies

The concept of a public health approach emerged in WHO as it recognised that the model of antiretroviral therapy (ART) delivery in well-resourced settings, specialist physician management and sophisticated laboratory monitoring, was not feasible in resource-poor settings. It was developed as work began on the "3x5" Initiative: pillar three emphasised simplified, standardised tools and user-friendly guidelines for delivering ART (World Health Organization (WHO), 2003b).

The term was originally used in 2002 as WHO published its first global guidelines "scaling up antiretroviral therapy in resource-limited setting: guidelines for a public health approach" (World Health Organization (WHO), 2002b). It was further developed in a short WHO monograph on the principles and practice of ART, where the common features of ARV programmes underway in developing countries were reviewed; and lessons drawn in overcoming constraints (World Health Organization (WHO), 2003a).

In 2006, WHO recognised that there was considerable uncertainty about what should constitute a public health approach to ART to enable access to treatment in developing countries to be scaled up and effectively delivered. The principles articulated in the 2002 guidelines and 2003 monograph were expanded and refined to clarify their relevance and importance for treatment providers, HIV programme managers and policymakers in developing countries. Conceptually, the approach took into account country requirements, the realities of weak health systems and the experiences of pioneering ART programmes. It dispelled concerns that ART guidelines successfully developed for resource-rich settings could not be adapted for resource-limited settings. The key elements of the public health approach to ART are outlined in Table 3.1 (Gilks et al., 2006).

The key tenets were the standardisation and simplification of ARV regimens to support efficient implementation, ensuring ART programmes were based on the most rigorous scientific data; and equity of ART delivery, aiming to set standards

DOI: 10.4324/9781003505693-5

Table 3.1 The key elements of the WHO public health approach to ART

Core principles	An equity and rights-based approach
	Universal access according to need
	One global standard of care
	Care and treatment free at the point of service delivery
Guidance to inform practice	Clear treatment goal – increased survival and quality of life
	Population-based rather than individual patient management
	Simplification and standardisation – regimens and formulations
	Simplification and standardisation – ART clinical management and decision-making
	Simplification and standardisation – parsimonious use of laboratory tests for clinical monitoring
	Global evidence-informed guidelines, regularly updated with new developments and scientific advances
Implementation	Hub and spoke district health model for decentralised and integrated service delivery
	Task shifting of clinical management actions to lower cadres
	ARV procurement: central purchasing and forecasting
	Simplified supply chains with linked to standardised management practices
	Simple medical records and registers to monitoring programme performance and product stock-keeping

for treatment that should be accessible by all in need. The key conceptual shift was the move from the individual patient to a population-based approach, recognised as the only way to make ART rapidly accessible to the millions in need.

The approach emphasised the centrality of delivering ART across the life-course; and clarified how clinical teams in primary care and second-level facilities were effectively enabled to deliver ART in resource-constrained settings. The term has continued to be used in all subsequent WHO guidelines, be they for HIV prevention, care, support or treatment, to highlight the continuing relevance of a public health approach in effecting global AIDS control. The single most innovative component was the concept of a first-line/second-line regime sequence for population-wide ART, in sharp contrast to the initial regimen a specialised physician would select and prescribe for their patient, subsequently changing ARVs according to the response to treatment in an individualised management approach. User-friendly practical guidelines made standardised recommendations for which ARV combinations should be made available and provided for free by the public health sector for first-line therapy; and when this failed what ARV medicines were reserved for second-line therapy in resource-limited settings.

Initially, there were three classes of antiretroviral medicines that were generally available and orally administered for the guidelines to consider: the nucleoside and non-nucleoside reverse transcriptase inhibitors (NRTIs and NNRTIs) and the protease inhibitors (PIs). More ARV classes have subsequently been developed, in particular the integrase inhibitors also known as integrase strand transfer inhibitors (INSTIs). In combination therapy, either a PI or an NNRTI (or latterly an INSTI) is anchored to an NRTI backbone, which usually has two different medicines making a triple ARV combination.

Physicians were uncertain which anchor drug to use for initial therapy in individualised patient management. NRTI/NNRTI combinations were widely used in Europe and North America as they were cheaper; with a lower pill-burden and less toxicity they were more tolerable and easier for patients to take. But equally many physicians prescribed PI-based therapy, citing potency and viral load response. With initial uncertainty, the first 2002 WHO ART guidelines made recommendations to consider all three classes of ARV medicines for both first-line and second-line ART. They were a start but were not particularly suited for ART scale-up.

Based on cost and availability, WHO made a pragmatic decision in 2006 to simplify the standardised recommendation for first-line ART to an NRTI/NNRTI combination; the option of triple NRTI therapy was never widely implemented. A wider set of WHO guidelines were released: revised guidelines for adult and adolescent ART (Gilks & Vitoria, 2006); new guidelines for treating pregnant women and preventing HIV infection in infants (World Health Organization (WHO), 2006a); and new guidelines for infants and children (World Health Organization (WHO), 2006c). All aimed to support universal access to ART according to need. Being pragmatic rather than evidence-based, this critical decision poorly aligned with "3by5" pillar five: rapidly identifying and reapplying new scientific knowledge.

The first trials of ART, all conducted in Industrialised settings, that showed ARVs were capable of halting and reversing HIV disease used clinical end-points (developing AIDS; mortality). But as highly effective combination therapy became standard of care far fewer clinical end-points developed and comparisons of different ARVs and ART regimens increasingly moved to use short-term surrogate markers of success. HIV can be measured in plasma; virus becomes undetectable with effective therapy but rises when therapy is failing, or the patient is non-adherent to treatment. It became the standard surrogate marker, and the goal of individualised ART has now become viral suppression.

The science behind these trials was important to guide physician preference but was difficult to interpret and problematic for evidence-based guidelines for developing country settings. Cost and availability were not considered. The "3by5" Initiative, and subsequent public health treatment programmes have always had as their goal prolonging survival and restoring quality of life with universally accessible ART. It was (and still is) unclear how short-term differences in viral load would play out long-term in either quality of life or overall survival. The costly technology to measure viral loads was not initially available in the public sector, nor was it likely to become widely accessible as ART was scaled up: purchasing and providing ARVs was the immediate priority. Hence, NRTI/NNRTI combinations were recommended for first-line ART. A further pragmatic and hard-headed decision was made to reserve the potent but more costly PIs for second-line ART.

Being prescriptive about first- and second-line treatment options allowed for the development of a simple formulary of anti-retroviral medicines which encouraged the production of fixed-dose first-line combinations with four two-drug, four three-drug and four co-packaged products available from at least 23 generic producers. This competition helped drive significant price reductions in low- and low-middle-income countries: depending on the regimen used, the price of first-line medicines decreased between 37% and 53%. In 2005 a fixed-dose adult combination first-line regimen with nevirapine as the NNRTI was available for US$148 per person per year. This in turn allowed much wider availability of treatment.

The fall in adult first-line drug pricing has been further fuelled by ongoing scale-up of treatment programmes as well as by increased competition among a growing number of products prequalified by WHO, and negotiations between the William J. Clinton Foundation (now the Clinton Foundation) and major generic manufacturers. The market and manufacturers were slower to respond to second-line and paediatric formulations, but substantial price reductions have nevertheless been achieved. Pricing has however remained relatively high in middle-income countries; and across the board most salvage therapy options are not discounted (World Health Organization (WHO), 2014a).

Simplified clinical decision-making and standardised monitoring

The second key aspect of the public health approach was that the clinician (initially a medically qualified practitioner, able to prescribe ART; latterly often a clinical officer or nurse-practitioner) did not have to decide what ARVs to use, much as a TB clinical officer does not decide which anti-tuberculosis medicines to use. They follow the guidelines and use the medicines that are provided for free in public sector dispensaries and pharmacies. This contrasted with individualised patient management where the specialist physician chose an initial regimen from the wide range of ARVs available in well-stocked public and private sector pharmacies; and changed ARV combinations for a variety of reasons: tolerability, drug-drug interactions, co-infections and viral load responses.

Simplified clinical management considered the critical decision-making steps, which often needed to be guided and informed by clinical monitoring without the benefit of routine laboratory monitoring. This was condensed down to the four S's: when to start ART; when to substitute one ARV for another ARV in the

Table 3.2 The four S's: simplified clinical decision-making for rolling out ART

Simplified clinical decision-making for ART based on a first-/second-line binary
When to *S*tart ART – guided by CD4 count and/or clinical monitoring When to *S*ubstitute within ARV class – guided by toxicity monitoring When to *S*witch to second-line for failure – guided by clinical monitoring and viral loads When to *S*top and move to end-of-life care – guided by patient preference

same class for toxicity management or co-infection treatment; when to switch for regime failure; and when to consider stopping for futility (Gilks et al., 2006) (Table 3.2).

When to start: in 2006 only 2 million persons in low- and middle-income countries were accessing treatment, making ART a limited good that had to be rationed for the sickest and most in need. Following HIV diagnosis, the decision when to start had to identify patients with the most advanced and severe HIV disease or AIDS, in need of immediate treatment.

Initial clinical assessment was mandatory for all newly diagnosed PLHA: Isoniazid preventive therapy and co-trimoxazole prophylaxis, to prevent TB and OIs, was recommended as an integral component of the HIV chronic care package and as a key element of pre-ART care (World Health Organization (WHO), 2006b). For those enrolled in care programmes, regular follow-up assessment was necessary to identify clinical deterioration and disease progression; and to support OI prophylaxis.

In settings with adequate resources, the CD4 count is routinely determined to establish a patient's degree of immunosuppression and over time the rate of destruction of the immune system. Plasma viral load is uninformative in the decision when to start ART. WHO revised its definitions for HIV surveillance and clinical and immunological staging of HIV-related disease in adults and children into four stages to support decision-making around ART. Presumptive and definitive criteria were established for HIV-related and AIDS-defining clinical staging events.

The consensus view was that any adult or adolescent with a CD4 count below 200 (immunological AIDS) should immediately start ART. There were more complex CD4-guided recommendations for infants and children. Many facilities however did not have access to laboratories that could measure CD4 counts or even total lymphocyte counts (a more widely available surrogate for CD4 count). Clinical staging alone was sufficient: stage 3 represented severe HIV-related disease and stage 4 was equivalent to AIDS and thus the need to start ART (World Health Organization (WHO), 2007d).

When to substitute within class: anti-retroviral medicines can be responsible for a wide range of toxicities, ranging from low-grade intolerance that may be self-limiting to life-threatening. Sick individuals and AIDS patients often have co-morbidities at the time of treatment initiation or that subsequently develop on ART and that need to be treated, with the risk of significant drug-drug interactions and the need to modify therapy accordingly. Tuberculosis is common in AIDS patients and can be particularly challenging to manage alongside ART. The 2006 guidelines developed standard definitions for grading and monitoring toxicity and drug-drug interactions; and standard operating procedures for their management.

The recommended approach was to try to identify the ARV medicine likely responsible for severe toxicity and/or drug-drug interactions; clearly differentiate this from first-line ART failure; and then to substitute the identified problem agent with another in the same ARV class. In practice it was possible to have one first-line regimen with just one or two substitute ARVs available. This simplified procurement and supply chain management, particularly if the alternate first-line regime was available in blister packs, co-packaged or co-formulated.

When to switch for failure: once a patient is commenced on first-line ART, regular clinical follow-up and assessment is important, supplemented if available by immunological or virological monitoring. Initial improvement followed by clinical deterioration, a fall in CD4 count or rise in plasma viral load requires careful assessment. The problem could be the absence of ARV medicines in the dispensary, a system failure with drug stockouts out of the individual's control; or it could be poor compliance with the patient not regularly taking their medicines and needing adherence support. These have to be differentiated from failing first-line therapy with the need to switch to second-line ART. Patient assessment includes history taking to check for poor adherence or medicine stockouts, physical examination and clinical staging to look for clear signs of deterioration towards stage 3 or stage 4, which strongly suggesting failure; and if available blood tests for CD4 count and plasma viral load.

The revised clinical staging and immunological classification of HIV-related diseases in adults and children provided updated guidance for clinical and immunological monitoring to identify treatment failure. One development was to recognise that clinical and immunological stage would significantly improve with effective ART before deteriorating with ongoing treatment failure. Previously AIDS surveillance and staging, developed prior to highly active ART, was hierarchical and irreversible: once a case, always a case of AIDS. Another development was to establish presumptive and definitive criteria for clinical staging events (World Health Organization (WHO), 2007d).

Because the decision to switch is such an important part of ART management, and also because second-line was much more expensive and less widely available than first-line therapy, many programmes opted to confirm failure with viral load testing or CD4 measurement, especially for infants and children. At the start of ART roll-out, the priority was to invest resources in purchasing medicines rather than expensive laboratory equipment, meaning that in practice access to plasma viral loads was very restricted. There was a trade-off between confirming failure then promptly switching to second-line; or continuing with a potentially failing first-line regimen thereby increasing the likelihood of drug resistance because of lack of access to virological monitoring.

When to stop: HIV treatment has been in general use in well-resourced settings for many years, initially with single drug monotherapy or relatively ineffective two drug combinations. Because HIV has a high mutation rate, HIV drug resistance (HIVDR) frequently emerges with ineffective therapy; a significant number of patients developed extensive drug resistance across most classes of ARV medicines rendering ART largely ineffective. Some patients opt to stop therapy with treatment fatigue and severe toxicity and move to end-of-life palliative care.

As ART scale-up was commencing in resource-limited settings with combination first-line, there was very little HIVDR: few patients had failed first-line or been non-compliant. The emergence of drug resistance was a real threat, and it was felt prudent to consider a time in the future when increasing numbers of patients were failing second-line therapy and consider their options. Simple assessment could identify second-line failure, exactly as for first-line: clinical staging, supplemented by CD4 and plasma viral loads. By analogy with cancer therapy, stopping for futility and moving to end-of-life care was one option. Equally well, if third-line ART therapy options ever became a realistic prospect, identifying second-line failure could trigger the switch to third-line, salvage therapy.

Monitoring and surveillance of HIV drug resistance: Rather than just waiting for the almost inevitable appearance and spread of HIVDR and considering how to manage its consequences, WHO developed a minimum-resource global strategy for prevention, surveillance and assessment of HIVDR (Bennett et al., 2008). It also established HIVResNet, a network of international experts to provide technical advice on activities to prevent, monitor and respond to HIV drug resistance; optimise the use of resistance testing; and support policies related to optimal first- and second-line ART selection (Bertagnolio et al., 2008). The Laboratory Network, a key subgroup, now includes more than 30 laboratories designated by WHO to perform quality-assured genotypic testing in order to support HIVDR surveillance in low- and middle-income countries.

Implementing population-wide public health ART

Population-wide implementation also needs simplified and standardised operational approaches. In tandem with the normative technical work involved in developing the public health approach, WHO developed the Integrated Management of Adolescent and Adult Illness, adapted from the Integrated Management of Childhood Illness (IMAI/IMCI) to facilitate decentralised implementation that is integrated within health systems. Practical tools and modules for service management, chronic HIV care with ARV therapy, training and job-aides for clinical teams, supportive supervision; patient education and self-management and a standard and simple patient-monitoring system were developed (World Health Organization (WHO), 2004a). These modules were the first to focus on the needs of first-level facility health workers where initial diagnosis and much of the long-term chronic care and treatment would be provided. They heralded a massive interest in and expansion of ways to promote integrated service delivery at the primary care level across the continuum of care.

Where the burden of HIV disease is high, health workers at the primary care level have a significant workload across a broad set of clinical tasks, including HIV testing and diagnosis, educating patients and carers to promote prevention, optimising retention in pre-ART care then managing ART. A linear cascade of care has conceptualised the steps through which patients must pass to be successfully treated: HIV testing; linkage to pre-ART care; ART initiation; retention in care.

The tasks involved with each step require different inputs and clinical skills. In view of the small number of doctors in most resource-constrained settings, and the concentration of specialists in cities, teams will have to largely rely on clinical officers, nurses and community health workers to deliver on these tasks. Task shifting, supported by the IMAI/IMCI approach, promotes the sharing of clinical management tasks and responsibilities to the lowest relevant cadre of health workers and then into the community, ultimately to engage the educated patients themselves.

Task shifting was a novel concept developed in the public health approach as a fundamental step to support chronic disease management and the shift to long-term treatment and care at the primary healthcare level. The need for task shifting was evident in high-burden HIV settings and IMAI/IMCI training and guidance modules supported its use. It was widely promoted by WHO and partners in ART scale-up despite the lack of an evidence-base to validate it. Out of necessity, some countries rapidly adopted it as a national policy and over time it has been generally taken up and widely used. Some tasks have been easier than others to shift: the need to be a qualified physician to initiate ART and sign repeat prescriptions was in some jurisdictions a legal issue as well as a service delivery issue; similarly, only a trained laboratory technician could perform HIV diagnostic testing and give out the results. Slowly these issues have been identified and largely overcome.

WHO with the support of PEPFAR and UNAIDS published recommendations and guidelines on task shifting which proposed the adoption or expansion of task shifting as a key method of strengthening and expanding the health workforce to rapidly increase access to decentralised HIV and other health services. Five key sets of recommendations were made: (a) to adopt task shifting as a public health initiative; (b) to create an enabling regulatory environment for implementation; (c) ways to ensure the quality of care; (d) ways to ensure sustainability; and (e) the organisation of clinical care services.

Task-shifting emerged from the programmatic endeavours to rapidly increase access to HIV services towards the goal of universal access. It was acknowledged that the impact of task shifting should not be restricted to HIV service delivery alone. The implications for other essential health services and the potential for wider health system strengthening were clear and emphasised. It was proposed as an efficient approach to help address the crippling health worker shortfall in many high-burden settings. However, substantial investments in human resources for health were, and still are required: task shifting cannot be a substitute for this (World Health Organization (WHO), 2007c).

The general adoption of the simplified, standardised recommendations for first-line ART and the falling costs of the ARVs greatly increased the volume of ARVs and other products to support care and treatment being shipped out to high-burden countries. Unfortunately, many countries had weak procurement and supply chains meaning that there were many delays and bottlenecks in the supply of ARVs in-country, from central medical stores and warehouses to the hospital pharmacies where they needed to be on the shelves if they were to be prescribed and dispensed. It was becoming clear that significant investments would be required to improve inefficient services and fragile supply chains. These were made as ART programmes gained momentum.

One further challenge was evident as the public health approach was implemented and ART roll-out proceeded at a pace: tracking the progress of patients on long-term treatment over time with no cure or end-point except loss-to-follow-up or death. It was relatively simple to count the numbers starting ART, and then using this to estimate ART coverage by country, region or globally. Keeping track of ART use at pharmacy or dispensing unit; clinical progress, including toxicity, interactions and ARV substitutions; and failure and ART regime switch to second-line, over time was more complex.

Using the example of TB control programmes, standard registers were developed with the potential to link with electronic medical records as they were developed. Regular register review enabled ARV use and future need to be quantified and linked with central medical stores for prompt ARV delivery to avoid drug stockouts; group cohort analysis provides core information for programme monitoring and evaluation, including outcome and survival. Tracking patients on ART as they returned to health and resumed economic activity was problematic if they moved districts; transfers out and in were complex to follow in a paper-based register system. Loss-to-follow-up for out-migration or other reasons, needed to be differentiated from death, but proved difficult.

The hub and spoke district health model for effective delivery of public health ART

The conceptual shift from individualised patient management to a public health population-based approach to ART was a fundamental enabler and key guiding principle for universal access to ART provided according to need in resource-limited settings. For reasons of both capacity and equity of access, the public health approach clearly recognised that to deliver ART at the population level, it was necessary to move beyond specialist tertiary hospitals and urban centres of excellence down to the health district and the primary care level serving rural, peri-urban and urban communities alike.

Decentralised services are core to the long-term effective delivery of ART at scale. Primary healthcare needs to be at the heart of this in order to achieve greater equity in access to healthcare, exactly as outlined in the Alma Ata declaration on primary healthcare of 1978 (Baum, 2007) and subsequently developed for HIV/AIDS in the MDGs by an exceptional focus and specific set of targets for ART (Ungurean, 2005). By itself however, primary healthcare cannot effectively deliver ART; hospital care need to be included and staff and clinical services integrated across the health district.

With treatment scale-up, ART and biomedical prevention is now mainly delivered outside large urban hospitals, beyond the traditional triangular hierarchy of care and is decentralised to the health district with clinical treatment teams usually headed by a trained physician but largely composed of clinical officers, nurses and community health workers and allied professions (pharmacists, laboratory technologists, counsellors, etc.) linked to community-based organisations and including people living with HIV, their families and lay providers. Task shifting has helped overcome some of the grave problems associated with a lack of human resources for health, particularly doctors, but across all cadres of health and allied workers. Using educated PLHA and lay providers makes an additional contribution at the community level.

The development of what some have called a hub and spoke model of district health services has been an important innovation for the decentralised delivery of ART and its effective scale-up: the hub is the district hospital, providing a variety of specialist services and housing the main pharmacy and district medical store; the spokes are the referral pathways from health centres, primary health clinics, community-based organisations and health posts to the hospital node and back down to the community and primary care level where most services are delivered (Abongomera et al., 2018) (Figure 3.1).

Physicians are usually based in the hub and depending on staffing levels and availability are posted out to large health clinics. Tasks are shifted within the hub to other clinicians, or from the hub to staff at the primary care facilities; patients move up and down the spokes. Clinical services need to be coordinated across the district: decentralisation is out from the hub to the peripheral facilities; medicines, diagnostics and supplies are ordered from the hub and delivered out via the spokes to primary care facilities according to their requirements. Supervisory visits should be made regularly from the hub to peripheral facilities but are often dependent on transport and vehicles.

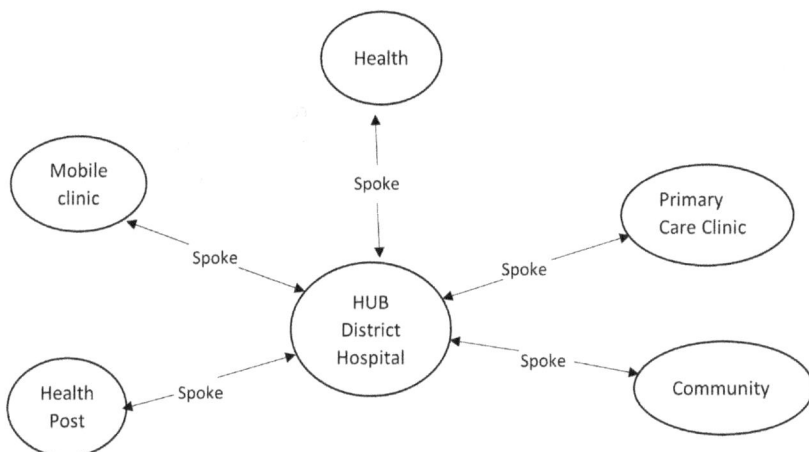

Figure 3.1 The hub and spoke model of the district health service for ART scale-up

The hub and spoke model facilitates the effective district-wide linkage of activities supporting those diagnosed with HIV to engage with prevention, care and treatment and support services as part of the continuum of HIV care. It also enables better retention of patients in care by ensuring there is continuity of service delivery between hospital and health clinic so that patients do not get lost in-between. A further key facet is the chance to incorporate ART into a broad range of services in particular ante-natal care and maternal and child health services and TB control services. Centrally-run vertical disease control programmes do not always find this easy to accomplish.

Better integrating HIV services has been key for the clinical teams, patients and their households. Integrated HIV health services are those managed and delivered in ways that ensures people receive a continuum of health promotion, disease prevention, diagnosis, treatment, disease management, rehabilitation and palliative care services at the different levels and sites of care within the health system, and according to their needs across the life-course. This sits well with the emerging concept of health services delivering people-centred HIV care. This consciously adopts the perspectives of individuals, families and communities in holistic ways; it needs people to have the education and support to make decisions and participate in their own care. It is organised around health needs and expectations of people rather than disease (World Health Organization (WHO), 2007b).

It is important to reflect on the person and patient journey as HIV/AIDS disease management and ART has evolved in low- and middle-income countries. As the epidemic started, the entry point to HIV/AIDS care was usually at tertiary or large second-level facilities: acutely sick AIDS patients often bypassed primary health clinics and presented directly to hospital. HIV was diagnosed; underlying co-morbidities treated; before ART, patients often died on the wards. With improvements in care and the rapid deployment of ART, the issue was to decongest specialist hospitals, to decentralise care to district hospitals and to integrate it with primary care. Effective integration was necessary as more and more patients commenced ART to avoid critical service overload.

Nowadays, when PLHIV fall sick, they are often still present directly to the nearest district hospital, where an initial diagnosis of underlying HIV or full-blown AIDS is made. Once the patient has been stabilised and entered a care programme or been started on ART, their long-term management has to be delivered at their nearest health centre or clinic by the primary healthcare team. Hospitals do not have the capacity to follow up each and every person on ART: services will collapse under the pressure and volume of work. Equally, if an individual is diagnosed when relatively well and starts HIV management at the primary care level, even with differentiated service delivery provision needs to be made for specialist consultation. Establishing referral pathways to a district hospital for physician or specialist review is important. But referral back to primary care when the problem is sorted is vital, to avoid congestion of hospitals. Hence the imperative for a hub and spoke district health model for effective delivery of ART and HIV care.

One criticism of Alma Ata and the primary care movement, and more recently people-centred healthcare, is that hospital-based disease-oriented care services are significantly down-played. AIDS is a complex clinical challenge, OIs and TB can prove difficult to diagnose and effectively treat; and ART is not always straightforward. By its very nature, effective delivery of ART has to incorporate hospital services and for equitable population-wide service delivery ensure effective integration with primary care services. ART and long-term clinical management of PLHA cannot be delivered and managed at the primary care level alone: more specialist hospital services need to be fully integrated.

Clearly, it is not an either-or binary nor a zero-sum game: it is both. Hence the importance of a hub and spoke district health model for effective public health ART biomedical prevention. This is the most effective place for the convergence of HIV with primary healthcare and its whole-of-society approach with three core components: primary care and essential public health functions as the core of integrated health services; multisectoral policy and action; and empowered people and communities (World Health Organization (WHO), 2023c).

4 Keeping the WHO public health approach fit for purpose

Updated goals and targets for a public health approach

As significant progress is made with antiretroviral therapy (ART) roll-out and more recently biomedical prevention, the context for goal and target setting has changed significantly. The first goals were mooted in the Millennium Declaration then set out in the millennium development goal (MDG) 6 to combat HIV/ AIDS along with malaria and other diseases and the targets: to have halted by 2015 and begun to reverse the spread of HIV/AIDS; to achieve by 2010 universal access to treatment for HIV/AIDS for all those who need it (United Nations (UN), 2000a).

This focussed down on ART in the "3by5" goal for WHO and partners to make the greatest possible contribution to prolonging the survival and restoring the quality of life of individuals with HIV/AIDS, advancing to the ultimate goal of universal access to ART for those in need of care, as a human right. The ambitious target was that by the end of 2005, 3 million eligible people in developing countries who need ART will be receiving effective ART (World Health Organization (WHO), 2003b).

Recognising the rapidly changing context for the global HIV response and the need to focus more on HIV prevention alongside ART delivery, UNAIDS developed a new strategic direction for the last five years of the MDGs boldly entitled "Getting to Zero": zero new infections; zero AIDS-related deaths; zero discrimination (Joint United Nations Programme on HIV/AIDS (UNAIDS, 2010). Much having being accomplished in the first decade, the 2011 update of the Political Declaration on HIV/AIDS upscaled the goal to eliminating HIV/AIDS as a public health threat and updated the number/date treatment target to "15by15" (United Nations (UN), 2011).

Following the 15-year MDG period, and learning many lessons from "3by5" and ART roll-out, a new set of much broader sustainable development goals (SDGs), were formulated and adopted by the UN to drive sustainable development in the next 15-year period to 2030 (Sachs, 2012). Of 17 inter-related goals, at least 10 are broadly concerned with health issues but only SDG 3 is specific to

DOI: 10.4324/9781003505693-6

health: ensuring healthy lives and promote well-being for all at all ages (Buse & Hawkes, 2015): the specific target for HIV/AIDS is now simply to end the epidemic of AIDS as a public health threat by 2030, with targets for other communicable diseases (TB, malaria, NTDs), non-communicable diseases (NCDs) and universal health coverage. The linkages provide an important framework for vertical disease control programmes to integrate with NCDs and to look forward towards UHC (Le Blanc, 2015).

UNAIDS developed three linked treatment targets to fast-track accelerated action to end the AIDS epidemic by 2030 (Joint United Nations Programme on HIV/AIDS (UNAIDS), 2015). They relate to three stages in the care continuum: the number of people living with HIV who know their status; among those who know their HIV status, the number who are accessing treatment; among those accessing treatment, the number who are successfully virally suppressed.

It is important not to regard these three discrete targets as a simple linear cascade of care. Clearly linked, the targets are nevertheless independent with different programmatic issues to overcome if they are to be achieved. The global targets were initially set in 2014 at 90-90-90, widely referred to as the three 90's. They reflected a fundamental shift in the approach to HIV treatment from the numbers accessing ART towards case detection, coverage and effective use of ART. They were reset in 2021 to 95-95-95 (Frescura et al., 2022).

In the spirit of what gets measured gets done, many target-specific indicators have been set across the SDGs. SDG target 3.3 is concerned with infectious diseases: by 2030, end the epidemics of AIDS, TB, malaria and neglected tropical diseases (NTDs) and combat Hepatitis, water-borne diseases and other communicable diseases. Indicator 3.3.1 is HIV incidence: the number of new HIV infections per 1,000 uninfected population by sex, age and key populations. There is no specific indicator for AIDS; adult and child AIDS deaths are generally used to measure progress towards ending AIDS by 2030. World Health Statistics is WHO's annual compilation of health-related data for member states. Since 2017, it has been titled "monitoring health for the SDGs" (World Health Organization (WHO), 2017b).

WHO guideline development: broadening scope and content

It is over 20 years since WHO first produced "Guidelines for a public health approach for scaling up ART in resource-limited settings" (World Health Organization (WHO), 2002b), and over 15 years since the 2006 landmark Lancet paper in which WHO set forth its vision for a public health approach to delivering ART, refining and expanding the key principles set out in 2002 and better articulating the foundations the public health approach established for ART scale up in resource-limited settings (Gilks et al., 2006). This articulation has been particularly important for ensuring that the WHO guidelines: recommendations for public health treatment kept abreast of the scientific advances in drug development and essential technologies, and programme experience of ART implementation.

In 2018, a review of the WHO public health approach to HIV treatment and care: looking back and looking ahead was published (Ford et al., 2018). This recognised that the approach had been broadly adopted in resource-limited settings and had provided the foundation for scaling up treatment to nearly 20 million people. It looked forward to the new global commitment to end the AIDS epidemic as a public health threat by 2030. It noted that the public health approach provided the necessary framework for guidelines to incorporate a wider scope of activities including counselling and testing, HIV prevention, comprehensive service delivery across the continuum of care, enhanced service delivery and programme monitoring as new targets were set as a pathway towards ending AIDS.

Over the last two decades, WHO guidelines have significantly evolved, been expanded in scope and consolidated over several domains: HIV prevention, testing, treatment, service delivery and monitoring. The guidelines are regularly revised and updated, following procedures established by the WHO guidelines review committee: new clinical and operational recommendations are based on the grading of recommendations, assessment development and evaluation (GRADE) approach; modelling studies, expert consultations and country case studies inform clinical, operational and programmatic guidance (World Health Organization (WHO), 2014b).

The different guidelines have incrementally included the scientific advances and implementation experiences across the several domains and have grown considerably in length and detail. They are detailed in Table 4.1. The most recent guidelines were published in 2021 and including annexes are now over 500 pages long (World Health Organization (WHO), 2021). All these guidelines and allied publications continue to make recommendations for a public health approach, which clearly has stood the test of time and remains as relevant today as it was in 2002.

The major scientific, clinical and programmatic advances since 2002 have been incorporated into the consolidated WHO guidelines under five separate but inextricably linked domains: combination prevention; HIV counselling and testing; ARV medicines; biomedical prevention; care and support; and service delivery. These are reviewed to highlight how flexible the public health approach framework has been as it has evolved to incorporate new knowledge and innovation to remain fit for purpose for HIV/AIDS programmes to meet new targets and goals.

It is important to appreciate this flexibility across one disease control programme as the approach is considered for complex chronic NCDs and other wicked health challenges facing resource-poor countries and communities. There are many common pathways that will be important as vertical programming

Table 4.1 Evolution of WHO guidelines for ART using a public health approach

Year published	Guideline title
2002	Scaling up ART in resource-limited settings: guidelines for a public health approach
2003 revision	Scaling up ART in resource-limited settings: treatment guidelines for a public health approach
2006	ART for HIV infection in adults and adolescents: recommendations for a public health approach
2006	Guidelines on co-trimoxazole prophylaxis for HIV-related infections among children, adolescents and adults: recommendations for a public health approach
2006 and 2007	Separate guidelines towards universal access for ART in infants and children and for antiretroviral drugs for treating pregnant women and preventing HIV infection in infants: recommendations for a public health approach
2007	Guidance on provider-initiated HIV testing and counselling in health facilities
2007	WHO case definitions of HIV for surveillance and revised clinical staging and immunological classification of HIV-related disease in adults and children
2010 revision	ART for HIV infection in adults and adolescents: recommendations for a public health approach
2010 revisions	Separate guidelines towards universal access for ART in infants and children and for antiretroviral drugs for treating pregnant women and preventing HIV infection in infants: recommendations for a public health approach
2011	Prevention and treatment of HIV and other sexually transmitted infections among men who have sex with men and transgender people: recommendations for a public health approach
2013	Consolidated guidelines on the use of antiretroviral drugs for treating and prevention HIV infection: recommendations for a public health approach
2016 second edition	Consolidated guidelines on the use of antiretroviral drugs for treating and prevention HIV infection: recommendations for a public health approach
2021	Consolidated guidelines on HIV prevention, testing, treatment, service delivery and monitoring: recommendations for a public health approach

The first 2002 guidelines had 67 pages; the 2021 Consolidated Guidelines had grown to 548 pages.

evolves with health systems strengthening to become horizontal, embracing integrated service delivery at district hospitals and primary healthcare level.

Combination prevention: know your epidemic, know your response

Understanding how the virus is transmitted and to whom is fundamental for the design of effective prevention strategies and their successful implementation. Initially these tended to be implemented individually; no stand-alone HIV prevention intervention is sufficient to control transmission and end the pandemic. One key advance has been the importance for countries to know your epidemic and your current response. This has come from the growing recognition that there is no single epidemic type but rather a multitude of diverse epidemics.

Combination prevention builds on the globally useful simple distinction between concentrated and generalised epidemics. Epidemics are concentrated if transmission occurs largely in defined vulnerable groups, now usually referred to as key populations: sex workers, men who have sex with men (MSM) and IDUs; and their sexual partners. Conversely, epidemics are generalised if HIV transmission is sustained by heterosexual behaviour in the general population and can readily be transmitted from mother to child (Wilson & Halperin, 2008).

Knowing your epidemic requires countries to identify the key drivers of ongoing transmission and their behavioural, social and structural promoters. Knowing your response enables countries to match and prioritise their response by identifying, selecting and funding those prevention measures that are the most appropriate and effective in relation to their specific epidemic scenarios and settings. Generally, interventions suitable for key populations have limited value in countries with generalised epidemics, though they may be critical if there are communities of MSM or IDUs. Interventions tailored for key populations will have little effect on women and do nothing to prevent mother-to-child transmission (Joint United Nations Programme on AIDS (UNAIDS), 2007).

Learning lessons from treatment, where different ARVs are combined for highly effective ART, as more options have emerged, so they have been combined to be more effective. Combination prevention programmes are rights-based, evidence informed and community-owned; and use a mix of biomedical, behavioural and structural interventions prioritised to meet the needs of individuals and communities so as to have the greatest sustained impact on reducing infections. They start with the basic construct of generalised or concentrated epidemics. Programmes are carefully tailored to national and local needs and conditions; focus resources on the strategic mix of programmatic and policy actions required to address documented risks and needs; and are planned and managed to operate synergistically, strategically and consistently over time and on multiple levels to address both immediate risks and underlying drivers of vulnerability (Hankins & de Zalduondo, 2010).

There are several examples in the literature outlining how countries have collected and analysed data and kept abreast of the growing number of data sources to better know their epidemic and then how to tailor an effective response. One describes how India has done this over a 15-year period as data sources expanded and the geographical units for data generation shifted from federal to state, district and then sub-district level. It also describes how standard analyses have informed an increasingly effective, well-targeted and decentralised national response (Sgaier et al., 2012).

Developments in HIV counselling approaches, HIV diagnosis and screening

As ART roll-out started in high-burden low-income settings, the public health approach recognised that the only laboratory result that was absolutely required for ART initiation was a positive HIV diagnostic test, ideally confirmed with a second test and accompanied by supportive HIV counselling. Informed consent was mandatory with pre-test counselling provided wherever possible. Counselling services were few and far between and based in urban areas. With limited laboratory capacity, HIV testing services (HTS) were often rudimentary; access was very limited, especially in rural areas.

Significant challenges existed: inefficient transport of blood samples to the laboratory and results back to the clinician ordering the test; widespread stigma and discrimination; and few trained counsellors. As a consequence, only some undertook HIV testing. When consent was given for testing, it could be weeks before a positive result was returned to the patient and the clinician: sick patients in hospital often died waiting for a result and there were long waiting times for post-test counselling services. On the wards, it was often assumed a sick AIDS patient had underlying HIV infection; in clinic, patients often had to make several visits until the result was reported back.

In a short 2004 policy statement on HIV testing, UNAIDS and WHO stipulated the "3 Cs" of HIV testing: confidential, accompanied by counselling and only conducted with informed consent. They distinguished four types of HIV testing: client-initiated voluntary counselling and testing (VCT) to learn HIV status and a critical entry point for prevention; diagnostic HIV testing, indicated whenever a person had signs and symptoms of HIV-related disease or AIDS; a routine offer of HIV testing by clinicians in STI clinics, in antenatal services drug use treatment services etc, in asymptomatic clients; and mandatory screening of blood or organ donors (UNAIDS & WHO, 2004).

Prior to the availability of highly effective combination ART, HIV testing was primarily client-initiated VCT with routine HIV screening of blood and blood products. A diagnosis of HIV was assumed in patients with clinical AIDS. There was limited use of co-trimoxazole (CTX) for OI prophylaxis and isoniazid preventative therapy (IPT) of TB. With significant stigma and discrimination, many opted not to be HIV tested. This reluctance became problematic as care services were being set up and ART was rolling out with a strong focus on equity: the reach of HTS was poor, with only 10% of those who needed VCT in low- and middle-income settings with access to counselling.

As ART became more widely available and pre-ART care including CTX and IPT was increasingly promoted, provider-initiated testing and counselling (PITC) approaches were advocated: healthcare workers and clinicians routinely initiate an offer of HIV testing in the context of effective HIV prevention or care services being available. In 2007, WHO issued guidance on PITC in health facilities. It urged health staff to recommend HIV testing and counselling as part of the standard of care to patients with signs of underlying HIV infection; and open this up to all patients attending a health facility in countries with generalised epidemics. It also included antenatal services and infants whose mother was known to have HIV infection (World Health Organization (WHO), 2007a).

Single-use rapid HIV tests are widely distributed to complement the standard multi-test laboratory approach using an enzyme immunoassay (EIA, often also called an ELISA test). A single EIA test costs less than a single rapid diagnostic test (RDT), but only when multiple tests are batched and done together. Where a large number of tests are regularly conducted, such as a busy district hospital with a working diagnostic laboratory, EIA testing is preferred. In settings where laboratory services are not readily accessible, an RDT is preferred: it can be carried out on the spot in the clinic and reported back within the hour. Showing the client the test result and the positive and or control lines in the test kit increases confidence with the result and if positive of their HIV diagnosis.

Resource and capacity constraints may require a phased implementation of expanded PITC services. Pre-test information can be provided to individuals particularly if an RDT is to be used; or to groups in health information talks, suited to situations like antenatal clinic waiting rooms, where large numbers of patients are to be offered EIA testing. Declining or opting out of an HIV test should not result in reduced quality of care or denial of services. Post-test counselling should link with HIV prevention services when the client is negative; and facilitate the entry into an ART programme and/or HIV care services if positive. Post-test counselling for pregnant women who test positive should also address birth plans, infant feeding options and infant and partner HIV testing.

In 2013, WHO released its first consolidated guidelines on ART for treating and preventing HIV infection: recommendations for a public health approach. They incorporated HIV testing as the entry point to prevention, care and treatment. All forms of testing and counselling remained voluntary and should adhere to the enlarged five C's outlined in Table 4.2. Verbal consent was regarded as sufficient, written consent was no longer required (World Health Organization (WHO), 2013).

WHO subsequently released guidance on service delivery including pre-test and post-test services; good practice for HTS; information on cost-effective approaches; HIV testing strategies and testing algorithms; quality assurance

Table 4.2 The five C's: guiding principles for HIV testing and counselling

The five C's	The key guiding principles
Consent	People receiving HIV testing and counselling must give informed consent for testing and counselling; and should be informed of the process and their right to decline. Verbal consent is sufficient and written consent is not required
Confidentiality	HIV testing and counselling services are confidential; results will not be disclosed without the consent of the person being tested. Although confidentiality is to be respected it should not be allowed to reinforce secrecy, shame or stigma
Counselling	Testing must be accompanied by appropriate pre-test information, which can be provided as group pre-test information; and followed up with high-quality post-test counselling
Correct test results	HIV testing providers should strive to provide high-quality testing services and quality assurance mechanisms should be in place to ensure the provision of correct test results
Connections to care	Connections to prevention, care and treatment services should include the provision of effective referral to appropriate follow-up services as indicated, including long-term prevention and treatment support

Mandatory or coerced testing from a health provider of partner is never appropriate.

of HIV testing results; and HIV testing in the context of surveillance. It recommended that trained lay health providers conduct HIV testing using RDTs in order to increase access to testing, particularly through community-based HTS. It also considered issues relating to HIV self-testing (HIVST), including approaches to introduce and monitor its acceptability, uptake and effectiveness (World Health Organization (WHO), 2015a).

Early treatment benefits the individual. With ART available to all PLHA in high-income settings, the focus is increasingly to identify those unaware of their HIV status. General population screening is recommended, with PITC and rapid HIV testing as part of routine healthcare. A systematic review of the cost-effectiveness of screening in high-income settings concluded the most effective option to be one-time screening of the general population together with annual screening of high-risk groups like injecting drug users (IDUs), female sex workers (FSW) or MSM (Bert et al., 2018). Despite the obvious advantages of population-wide HIV screening in countries with generalised epidemics, few have taken this on: cost and capacity are major constraints.

In many high- and middle-income countries, RDTs are now readily available over the counter in retail pharmacies and other outlets. The opportunities for

HIVST have greatly increased and the paradigm for HIV testing as the first step in the care continuum has shifted. HIVST is widely promoted as a key development to support regular HIV testing in high-risk groups, particularly FSW or IDUs who may irregularly attend facilities where HTS services are available. In many countries where HIV has unfortunately crossed the boundaries of sexual orientation, gender, age and ethnicity, risk-based testing can fail to identify many people with HIV (McGuire et al., 2021).

WHO recommends HIVST as an additional approach that complements and creates demand for existing services and has developed a guide for planning introducing and scaling it up particularly in low-income settings where there is significant shortfall in HIV testing. It considers that HIVST can contribute to filling gaps in HIV programmes by reaching people with high HIV risk and vulnerability who have not tested; by creating demand for HIV prevention for those who test negative; by improving testing coverage through integrating HIVST in clinical services where HIV testing is needed but not routinely provided; and by facilitating partner testing, an effective but often underutilised testing approach (World Health Organization (WHO), 2018).

Advances with ARVs for treatment: new classes, products and formulations

As ART was rolled out in the global south, combination therapy was already widely available and used in high-income settings. Physicians had the choice of many oral antiretrovirals from three major classes of medicines: the NRTIs, the NNRTIs and the PIs. Two other classes – the entry inhibitors and fusion inhibitors – were rarely used, most often for salvage therapy in patients with extensive drug resistance. In the public health approach, the standardised recommendation for first-line ART was an NRTI/NNRTI combination: PIs were reserved for second line supported by recycled NRTIs. The simplified first-line, second-line binary has stood the test of time: millions have benefited from ART, prices have significantly dropped and rural as well as urban communities have had access to primary healthcare and hospital services to support its delivery.

Modified medicines in the NRTI class, nucleotide rather than nucleoside reverse transcriptase inhibitors, are now widely available along with less toxic and better tolerated NRTIs. They have been incorporated into public health ART guidelines and extensively deployed in resource-limited settings. The best example is the wholesale substitution of stavudine (d4T) by other NRTIs, particularly zidovudine (AZT) or tenofovir (TDF) to avoid highly stigmatising lipodystrophy and lipoatrophy. A new type of NRTI, the transcriptase translocation inhibitors, is under development. Islatravir is the first-in-class and has multiple mechanisms of action but adverse side effects that may limit its use.

In the NNRTI class, efavirenz has largely replaced the cheaper but more toxic nevirapine, with co-formulated tenofovir-lamivudine-efavirenz (TLE) becoming the preferred and most widely used single tablet drug combination in resource-limited settings. In industrialised setting the more costly second-generation oral NNRTI rilpivirine is favoured by many physicians, largely because it better retains activity in the face of HIV drug resistance. Dapivirine (DPV) has been developed particularly as a microbicide for HIV prevention.

One major new ARV class has emerged as a game changer in the last 20 years: the integrase inhibitors, also known as integrase strand transfer inhibitors (INSTIs). Raltegravir, the first-in-class, was licenced for use in the US in 2007; dolutegravir, elvitegravir and then bictegravir followed. Second-generation INSTIs are in development or in use: cabotegravir is the most evaluated investigational agent. The INSTIs target a distinct step in the retroviral life cycle and have been widely used in Industrialised setting as the anchor drug in initial therapy, or in highly-treated individuals with drug resistance.

Because of high rates of NNRTI resistance, dolutegravir has been widely used in low-income settings in first-line therapy. Together with two NRTIs tenofovir and lamivudine, dolutegravir is available as a co-formulated single tablet drug combination, often referred to as TLD. In a major development, WHO guidelines now recommend TLD as the preferred first-line single tablet regimen for initiating ART. The transition to TLD is now underway, but some countries still continue to prefer and provide TLE as their standard single tablet first-line regimen. WHO consider this an alternative first-line regimen (World Health Organization (WHO), 2021).

In second-line ART, ritonavir-boosted lopinavir and darunavir (with an optimised NRTI backbone) have become the most widely used PIs as they are better tolerated and do not need multiple dosing; significant drug-drug interactions with antituberculosis medicines, especially rifampicin, remain a challenge with the ritonavir boost. Dolutegravir can be used as the preferred second-line anchor drug with optimised NRTIs when TLE is the failing first-line regimen; patients can also safely substitute dolutegravir for ritonavir-boosted PIs (Paton et al., 2021). Boosted PIs with optimised NRTIs are recommended as a preferred second-line when TLD is the failing first-line regimen.

A further novel type of ARV medicines, the capsid inhibitor class, is under active development by the pharmaceutical industry. These molecules target the capsid shell of the virus and can be used to treat extensively drug-resistant infections. Lenacapavir is the first-in-class and is highly potent with a long half-life allowing oral dosing daily to weekly. It is being evaluated for use in initial therapy and in individuals with extensive treatment experience and multi-class drug resistance.

These new drug classes and second-generation NRTIs and NNRTIs have opened up the possibility of third-line ART options when second-line is failing. WHO recommends national programmes to develop policies for third-line ART, and make a conditional recommendation that they should include new drugs with minimal risk of cross-resistance to previously used regimens, such as an INSTI or second-generation NNRTIs and PIs (World Health Organization (WHO), 2021).

There has also been intense research and development into long-acting (LA) formulations for treatment. These can be administered orally or parenterally by injection, microneedle skin patches or implantable formulations. Reducing the frequency of administration, to monthly or bi-monthly dosing, may improve adherence and increase patient satisfaction by reducing visits to health facilities to pick up medicines (Nachega et al., 2023). The molecules being developed for long-acting formulations include cabotegravir (CAB), rilpivirine (RPV), lenacapavir and islatravir.

Large-scale trials of CAB/RPV LA have demonstrated non-inferiority of monthly and two-monthly injections with standard oral ART and it is now the first complete combination regimen to be licenced and recommended for initial treatment in high-income settings (Swindells et al., 2020). High costs may initially limit CAB/RPV use in low- and middle-income settings. Lenacapavir has also been licenced but only for treatment of patients with extensive treatment experience and multi-class drug resistance. Modelling suggests that CAB/RPV LA may have a role in sub-Saharan Africa if targeted to people with poor adherence but a recent review noted that data from clinical trials are needed to inform policy about LA first-line regimens in low-income settings (Cresswell & Lamorde, 2022).

Long-acting monoclonal antibodies (MABs) for immunotherapy are in the investigational pipeline; all need to be parenterally administered. Ibalizumab has already been approved in the US for use in combination with optimised ART; leronlimab is an investigational CCR5 antagonist. This approach is likely only to be available in tertiary hospitals under strict specialist supervision, and is not likely to be part of the public health approach in resource-limited setting anytime soon because of the cost and complexity of administration (Cresswell & Lamorde, 2022).

Unlocking antiretroviral medicines for biomedical prevention

In the early 1990s, a landmark clinical trial carried out by the Paediatric AIDS Clinical Trials Group established that zidovudine (a widely used ARV in the NRTI class) could greatly reduce maternal-infant HIV transmission (Connor et al., 1994). The PACTG trial was complimented by studies in West Africa that showed a short regimen of zidovudine was effective and tolerable to reduce vertical transmission of HIV in breastfed children (Dabis et al., 1999); and in Thailand that showed shortened zidovudine regimens could prevent mother-to-child HIV transmission (Lallemant et al., 2000). These studies were the first to demonstrate the impact that ARVs could have in biomedical prevention.

Mother-to-child transmission is the most important source of HIV infection in children. In 2001, the UN committed to reducing the proportion of infants infected with HIV by 20% by 2005 and by 50% by 2010 (United Nations (UN), 2001). WHO convened a technical consultation on ARVs and the prevention of mother-to-child transmission (PMTCT) in 2004 then published recommendations for a public health approach for ARVs to treat pregnant women and prevent HIV infection in Infants, towards universal access (World Health Organization (WHO), 2006a). Note that India and other countries prefers to refer to the prevention of parent to child transmission to ensure that it is not the mother alone who is seen as responsible and to blame for infant HIV infection.

Post-exposure prophylaxis (PEP) to protect healthcare workers who have had a needle-stick injury potentially contaminated with HIV-infected blood was the other initial way ARVs were used to prevent HIV transmission. Disease prophylaxis has also long been a mainstay of pre-ART care. Tuberculosis preventive therapy can substantially reduce the risk of active TB in PLHIV; WHO recommends IPT for six months in adults. Uptake is variable in settings with high prevalence of HIV and TB: national campaigns can substantially increase IPT use (Musaazi et al., 2023). Similarly CTX prophylaxis is of proven benefit in preventing a wide range of HIV-related opportunistic infections in adults (Suthar et al., 2015) and in infants and children (Chintu et al., 2004).

Combination HIV prevention recognises that no single prevention strategy is sufficient to control the pandemic. Yet somehow biomedical interventions were slow to be incorporated into rights-based combination prevention that favoured behavioural and structural approaches for addressing risk and vulnerability. A comprehensive approach clearly needs to tackle structural barriers that reduce the ability of individuals and communities to protect themselves against HIV infection (Hankins & de Zalduondo, 2010). But these approaches alone are insufficient particularly in countries with generalised epidemics and where infant infection is most prevalent.

Designing the optimal package of interventions needs to match the epidemiological profile of the population or region. It is critical to consider ARV medicines, along with a growing number of other effective biomedical or biobehavioural interventions like behavioural change, condom use, male medical circumcision particularly in Southern and Eastern Africa and needle exchange in drug using communities in combination prevention (Kurth et al., 2011). Two recent programmatic innovations have emphasised this: antiretroviral treatment as prevention (TasP), also known as test and treat (T&T); and using ARVs for pre- or post-exposure prophylaxis.

The core premise in TasP is that the lower the viral load is in an individual on ART, the lower the risk of onward HIV transmission (Quinn et al., 2000). A defining modelling study in 2009 asked how most effectively to deploy ART as a strategy to eliminate HIV in South Africa: universal voluntary HIV testing with immediate ART for those found positive could greatly accelerate the transition from endemic HIV to an elimination phase; and reduce the incidence to less than one person per 1000 people per year within five years (Granich et al., 2009).

Major trials provided the evidence base: the HPTN 052 study of discordant couples demonstrated that the early initiation of ART led to a sustained (>90%) reduction in HIV transmission to linked partners (Cohen et al., 2016); the Pop-ART study of universal testing and treatment in communities in Southern Africa showed that a combination prevention intervention with ART resulted in a 30% lower HIV incidence of infection than standard care alone (Hayes et al., 2019).

Sustaining high ART coverage through population-level TasP and in some countries universal testing and treating prompted the earlier initiation of ART in many jurisdictions and is widely credited with accelerating the reduction of HIV incidence globally. From the individual perspective, TasP means that with an undetectable viral load on ART the virus cannot be sexually transmitted. Scientists and the Prevention Access Campaign launched the Undetectable=Untransmissible (U=U) initiative (Eisinger et al., 2019). The science of treatment as prevention may not be widely understood by people and communities who would benefit from this information. Improving knowledge and attitudes towards U=U is likely to realise beneficial impacts on stigma, HIV prevention, testing and retention in care (Calabrese & Mayer, 2020).

The core premise with HIV prophylaxis is that if ARVs are present in the body around a potential transmission event, the virus will be inactivated and prevented from establishing infection in the exposed individual. PEP has been available in hospital settings for health professionals following needle-stick exposure for decades: AZT then various ARV combinations have been used. More recently it has been used by individuals post high-risk sex. PEP needs to be started very soon (within 48–72 hours) after exposure to be effective.

Pre-exposure prophylaxis (PrEP) as the name suggests necessitates having ARVs present in the blood or locally (for vaginal or anal sex) before the exposure event. A variety of delivery mechanisms have been developed and evaluated: the oral route for ARV pills; injectable long-acting formulations; and topical microbicide gels or vaginal rings impregnated with ARVs. There is strong evidence of PrEP effectiveness (Celum & Baeten, 2020). High-risk individuals are the target for and main users of PrEP, in particular gay and bisexual men who have sex with men (GBMSM), transgender women and men, sex workers, and particularly in Southern Africa young women.

A WHO policy brief in 2015 recommended people at substantial risk of HIV should be offered oral PrEP containing TDF (World Health Organization (WHO), 2015b). Australia has shown how effective daily oral PrEP can be at the community level in a situation of universal healthcare, subsidised PrEP and high health literacy (Grulich et al., 2021). The roll-out and global population-level effects of once-daily oral PrEP have fallen short of its potential: access to PrEP is far from universal; many individuals who start it discontinue quickly, while those who persist struggle to take a pill every day (Haberer, Mujugira, & Mayer, 2023). PrEp is also highly effective when used "on-demand", immediately before and after sex; this approach is now used is some countries (Molina et al., 2017).

Reliance upon male-controlled methods like condoms or male medical circumcision offers women limited power and agency to manage their own HIV protection. Vaginal microbicides offer a female-controlled biomedical intervention for preventing HIV. Several different microbicides have been evaluated, as gels or implanted into rings; some have general microbicidal activity, others have included ARV molecules. A thorough systematic review and meta-analysis found that the long-acting intravaginal ring containing dalpivirine significantly reduced risk of HIV transmission by 29%; the remaining microbicides had no evident effect (Musekiwa, Fernando, & Abariga, 2020).

Injectable long-acting ARV formulations offer a new, additional option for biomedical prevention in people at substantial risk of acquiring HIV, potentially overcoming some of the obstacles in uptake, adherence and retention seen with oral PrEP. They have generated much interest. Recent trial data has shown the safety, efficacy and acceptability of CAB-LA and many see this as a potential game-changer in HIV prevention. There are some obstacles to overcome, including high cost, complexity of administration and follow-up, and break-through infections before it can achieve its full potential (Liegeon & Ghosn, 2022). Islatravir is another long-acting ARV but recent safety concerns with high doses for treatment have put on hold PrEP studies and the development of injectable formulations.

Boosting HIV/AIDS service delivery at the district level

There have been several developments to broaden access to care and sustain service delivery at the district level as pressures mount on providers with more and more patients on ART and increasing demand for biomedical prevention interventions. These include when to start ART; monitoring the response to ART; improving retention in care; managing advanced HIV disease; integrating NCDs into the service package; and driving impact through programme monitoring and management. These have incrementally been included in updates of the WHO consolidated guidelines and helped to keep the public health approach fit for purpose. Recently there has also been a pressing need to cope with the pressures imposed on fragile health services by the SARSCoV2/COVID-19 pandemic.

When to start ART: As ART has become generally available it has ceased to be a rationed good in short supply, prioritised for the sickest and those in greatest need as assessed clinically or a CD4 count below a 200 threshold. Several studies have critically looked at the optimal time to initiate treatment, balancing adverse events, adherence, drug resistance and cost with reduced morbidity and improved survival. Following the SMART study, the CD4 threshold was generally agreed to be below 350 (Strategies for Management of Antiretroviral Therapy Study Group, 2008). Subsequently, the START study concluded that initiation of ART above a CD4 500 threshold study provided net benefit (Insight Start Study Group, 2015) although long-term follow-up showed the benefits rather diminished over time (INSIGHT Strategic Timing of AntiRetroviral Treatment Study Group, 2023).

This high-quality evidence base has led WHO to recommend universal treatment: ART should be initiated in all people living with HIV regardless of clinical stage and CD4 count as soon as possible after diagnosis. The "treat all" policy, as it has come to be known, is fully congruent with population-level TasP/T&T approaches for biomedical prevention and presents strategic opportunities for health systems to further reduce both HIV incidence and AIDS mortality. Most countries have adopted the "treat all" policy despite implementation challenges, capacity limitations and cost constraints.

Monitoring the response to ART: Once treatment is initiated, it is important regularly to monitor the individual for signs and symptoms of ARV toxicity, which necessitates an in-class drug substitution; and for treatment response necessitating a switch to second-line when failure is detected. Clinical monitoring by itself is a crude indicator of treatment failure but is universally applicable in primary care as well as in hospital settings. CD4 counts have some role in detecting failure when they fall after rising on initiation of effective treatment. The best way to identify treatment failure is with viral load testing; detectable virus is an indication of either poor adherence or a failing regime. It is always important to exclude poor adherence before concluding first-line therapy is failing.

The main problem with routine viral load testing is the limited accessibility of laboratories equipped with the technology to perform the test. Often samples have to be sent to a district centre with long turn-around times for results to be returned. Innovations like dried blood spots directly collected on filter paper, particularly useful for early infant diagnosis in PMTCT programmes, cannot overcome the need to send samples to a remote laboratory. While HIVDR testing is standard practice in high-income settings, it is clear that there is no role for individual HIVDR testing to manage treatment failure to guide choice of second-line ART in public health ART (Siedner et al., 2021).

Improve retention in care: With increasing numbers of people initiated on ART through treat all policies, gaps in service provision are likely to shift from access to treatment to long-term engagement with care as the key modifiable mediator of treatment success. Because the cascade of care identifies sequential steps in the care pathway and the numbers at each stage, it permits analysis of patient behaviour in the interval between diagnosis and sustaining long-term ART, for monitoring patient engagement and for targeting interventions to improve retention of those transitions with greatest attrition.

Care cascade research has helped quantify patient losses, identify the steps with greatest attrition and target interventions to improve retention in care. Before the treat all era, there was significant attrition during pre-ART care, with patients regularly needing review until they fulfilled eligibility criteria to start ART. With immediate or rapid initiation of ART, this part of the cascade is

Table 4.3 The cyclical cascade of care

Stage in the cyclical HIV cascade	Definition
Stage 1: HIV diagnosis; or re-diagnosis if disengaged from cascade after testing	The interval from receiving a positive HIV test to enrolling in an HIV treatment programme as a new or returning client
Stage 2: Linked to care; or relinked to HIV care if disengaged after initial linkage	The interval from enrolling in an HIV treatment programme as a new or returning patient to receiving the first ART dose
Stage 3: Initiated on ART; or reinitiated on ART if disengaged from ART services	The interval from the first ART dose to initial viral load test and retention on therapy
Stage 4: early retention: for first six months	Early retention to first 6-month viral load test
Stage 5: long-term retention: 6 months or more	Long-term retention until disengagement (30 days or more without ART) or death

The definitions assist research and in ART monitoring and evaluating ART programme performance.

becoming redundant. A cascade that better encompasses the complex cycle of engagement, disengagement, temporary disruptions, re-engagement and transitions in the care continuum has recently been developed (Ehrenkranz, Rosen, et al., 2021) (Table 4.3).

High retention has been achieved in streamlined HIV care delivery in the context of universal test-and-treat (Brown et al., 2016). Community-based interventions result in higher rates of treatment engagement and at least similar levels of retention in care and clinical outcome compared to facility-based care models (Nachega et al., 2016). WHO recommends that programmes should provide community support and interventions, such as adherence clubs and extra care for high-risk people to improve retention in HIV care; and implement interventions to trace people who have disengaged from care and provide support for re-engagement (World Health Organization (WHO), 2021).

Differentiated service delivery (DSD) is a patient-centred approach that simplifies and adapts HIV services across the care cascade in ways that serve the needs of the person, promotes retention in care and critically can significantly reduce unnecessary burdens on the health system. It can be effectively linked with patient-centred care for PLHIV (Ehrenkranz et al., 2021). Well-known models have focussed on ART delivery to patients who are clinically stable with little requirement for regular facility attendance but still need sustained ART. Existing evidence suggests that retention in care in DSD models are equivalent to conventional care (Long et al., 2020). A client-based model that provides tiered needs-based care tailored to the individual's requirements allows healthcare resources to be targeted to those with the greatest need or minimised when the client is stable only requiring a repeat prescription (Grimsrud et al., 2016).

Management of advanced HIV disease: In adults, adolescents and children older than five years, advanced HIV disease is defined as CD4 count below 200 and/or having WHO stage 3 or 4 disease; all children below five are considered to have advanced disease. A significant number, approaching 30% in some low- and middle-income settings present for care and start ART with advanced HIV disease. An additional number with advanced HIV disease have interrupted ART and are re-engaging with care when sick. At the individual level, those presenting with advanced HIV disease are at higher risk of death, even after starting ART; at the health system level, advanced disease is associated with increased healthcare costs. Nevertheless, it is clear that adults with advanced disease do respond very well to ART once it is started, with five-year survival over 90% (DART Trial Team, 2010).

The leading causes of morbidity and mortality in patients with advanced HIV disease in low- and middle-income countries include TB, severe bacterial infections and cryptococcal meningitis. The classic AIDS-defining OIs and cancers that are well recognised in high-income settings are of less importance. There are two priorities for the care of people with advanced disease: a package of care that covers the main causes of advanced HIV disease; and quickly starting the patient on first-line ART. WHO has produced guidelines for managing advanced HIV disease and rapid initiation of ART (World Health Organization (WHO), 2017a). A recent viewpoint has emphasised that ending AIDS deaths requires significant improvements in clinical care for people with advanced HIV disease who are seriously unwell when they present for care (Burke et al., 2023).

Integrating NCDs into the service package: People living with HIV are at increased risk of NCDs, especially cardiovascular disease, cervical cancer, diabetes and mental health conditions. Some of this risk is directly attributed to HIV, some relates to long-term drug toxicity and some relates to lifestyle. With increased coverage of ART and earlier initiation of therapy, the life expectancy of PLHIV has significantly improved (Autenrieth et al., 2018), exposing individuals to the risk of diseases common with ageing through longer exposure to standard NCD risk factors. Providing HIV care across the continuum creates an opportunity to assess, monitor and manage NCDs in PLHIV, especially in primary care settings. Integrating interventions for the prevention and management of NCDs in HIV services can reduce the risks of NCDs among PLHIV and contribute to sustaining the survival gains with long-term ART.

As a start, WHO has recently outlined strategic actions and practical solutions for integrating NCD services into other programmes and broader health systems, as appropriate and relevant to country context. The objective of the implementation guidance is to maximise the impact of health services and extend access to NCD care; it focusses on integrating the prevention and control of NCDs in HIV/AIDS, TB and sexual and reproductive health (SRH) programmes into primary healthcare at national, subnational and local levels (World Health Organization (WHO), 2023a).

WHO has also identified NCD actions and services to be prioritised and integrated into HIV service packages: the prevention, early detection and management of hypertension, diabetes and cardiovascular diseases; and screening and treatment of pre-cancerous lesions to prevent cervical cancer. It has also outlined approaches and actions to promote integration of NCD services into HIV services (World Health Organization (WHO), 2023b). These fit nicely with the recommendations for managing common coinfections and comorbidities, which includes NCDs, in the current 2021 consolidated guidelines.

Driving impact through programme monitoring and management: Monitoring and evaluation help programme managers assess the effectiveness and uptake of interventions for HIV prevention and establishes links between services along the cascade of care. Robust and actionable information is essential to identify gaps and bottlenecks in ART programme performance and to respond to them. Patient monitoring systems that link with one another are needed to track people receiving care as they move between clinics and districts over time and to ensure retention in care. As programmes mature, monitoring of individual- and national-level outcomes, including new HIV diagnoses, ART coverage, viral suppression, mortality, survival, ARV toxicity and adverse events and the emergence and transmission of HIV drug resistance become increasingly important to assess the quality and impact of programmes, and to further contribute to their optimisation over time.

Recently, WHO has updated its consolidated strategic information guidelines to provide a revised set of aggregate indicators and guidance on choosing, collecting and systematically analysing strategic information to manage and monitor the national health sector response to HIV. The indicator set is summarised in Table 4.4 and represents the current state of the response. The guidelines seek to support programme managers identify and close gaps in service access, coverage and quality across the HIV service cascade and continuum of care, from primary prevention to knowing one's HIV status to viral suppression (World Health Organization (WHO), 2020)

Table 4.4 Recommended top national core indicators according to programme domains

Strategic objective	Programme domain	National priority indicator
Reduce new infections among those at substantial risk	Condoms	# Condom use (key and general populations)
	PrEP	# PrEP uptake
	Other prevention	# Coverage of HIV prevention in key populations
		# Needles and syringes distributed

(Continued)

Table 4.4 (Continued)

Strategic objective	Programme domain	National priority indicator
95% of PLHIV know their status and are linked to treatment	HIV Testing Services	# PLHIV who know their HIV status # HIV testing volume and positivity # Linkage to ART
95% of PLHIV identified on ART and 95% on ART virally suppressed	ART and viral loads	# PLHIV on ART # Total attrition from ART # PLHIV who have suppressed viral loads
Reduce TB mortality	TB/HIV	# TB preventive therapy initiation # Completion of TB preventive therapy
Reduce new infections among children	Vertical Transmission	# Viral suppression at labour and delivery # Early Infant Diagnosis coverage
Reduce co-morbidity and mortality of STIs	Sexually Transmitted infections (STIs)	# Syphilis screening and treatment coverage # Cervical cancer screening in women with HIV
Zero HIV discrimination	Stigma	# Avoidance of healthcare due to Stigma and Discrimination in key populations

5 Ending AIDS and planning for endemic HIV

Exceptional progress with controlling HIV/AIDS in the global south

Since the 2001 UNGASS Declaration of Commitment on HIV/AIDS, truly remarkable achievements have been made with the equitable scaling up of antiretroviral therapy (ART) to those in need of treatment and delivery of combination prevention to communities at risk of HIV. Few would have predicted such progress and programmatic success across the global south in just two decades of an exceptional response backed up by specific funding mechanisms and guided throughout by a public health approach. Nor how the responses developed to combat AIDS would help shape and define the global health movement.

Global HIV and AIDS statistics are reported annually by UNAIDS in the annual global AIDS update (Joint UNAIDS Programme on HIV/AIDS (UNAIDS), 2023). Four significant achievements stand out:

- *Progress with delivering ART*: From a very low base in 2002 as "3×5" started, when less than 400,000 people in resource-limited settings were estimated to be on ART, to 29.8 million people accessing ART by the end of December 2022. ART coverage in sub-Saharan Africa, the continent bearing the brunt of the AIDS epidemic, was just 2% in 2002; global ART coverage had reached 76% by December 2022 (95% confidence intervals (CIs) 65–89).
- *Declines in AIDS deaths*: By the end of 2022, annual AIDS-related deaths have been reduced by 69% to around 650,000 (CIs 510,00–860,000) since the global peak in 2004 when around 2 million (CIs 1.6–2.7 million) were estimated to have died.
- *Reductions in numbers newly infected with HIV*: An estimated 1.3 million (CIs 1.0–1.7 million) people became newly infected with HIV in 2022, a 57% reduction since global HIV incidence peaked in 1996.
- *Impact of PMTCT programmes*: in 2022, 82% (CIs 64–98%) of pregnant women living with HIV had access to ARVs to prevent transmission to their child. Since 2010, when programmes started to be significantly ramped up,

DOI: 10.4324/9781003505693-7

new infections among children have declined by 58% from 310,000 (CIs 210,000–490,000) to 130,000 (CIs 90,000–210,000) in 2022.

These achievements mean that by the end of 2022, 39 million people globally were estimated to be living with HIV, up from just under 30 million PLHIV in 2000. Prevalence has continued to rise, even as incidence has significantly dropped – a cause for alarm for some policymakers when told of programmatic successes; and sometimes confusion for students. There is a simple explanation for this seeming epidemiological paradox: HIV is a fatal disease; successful treatment prevents AIDS deaths but does not cure infection, meaning that prevalence, the number of people on ART living with chronic HIV, inexorably rises.

Achievements in reaching the 90-90-90, now 95-95-95 targets are helpful to monitor global progress towards the goal of ending HIV/AIDS as a public health threat by 2030. In 2022, 86% PLHIV knew their status; among those who knew their status, 89% were accessing treatment; and among people accessing treatment, 93% were virally suppressed.

Recognising that 200 cities and municipalities globally account for 60% of people living with HIV and that most low- and middle-income countries are rapidly urbanising, UNAIDS with partners set up a network of Fast-Track Cities pledging to attain and surpass 90-90-90 targets and end urban HIV by 2030. By the end of 2019, over 300 cities had joined: one had achieved 95-95-95; four had achieved 90-90-90 and 34 had achieved one or two of the targets (Duncombe et al., 2019).

Global numbers miss some granularity, particularly at the country level. A recent paper has noted what has been achieved by PEPFAR in Uganda, the first country to set up a PEPFAR programme back in 2004. In collaboration with other stakeholders and the Government of Uganda, by September 2022 more than 1.3 million people were receiving ART, a 5000% increase from programme inception; ART scale-up averted an estimated 600,000 deaths and prevented 500,000 infections; mother-to-child-transmission rates decreased over 70% from 6.4% in 2010 to 1.5% in 2022. Viral load was suppressed in 95% of adults and 85% of children on ART in 2022 (Dirlikov et al., 2023).

Decades of successful ART have translated into significant survival benefit: in Europe and North America, for people with HIV who started ART with high CD4 counts, life expectancy is only a few years lower than for the general population; estimates are substantially lower in people with low CD4 counts at ART initiation, emphasising the continued importance of early diagnosis and rapid initiation of treatment (Trickey et al., 2023).

Globally, this has meant that the number of PLHIV over the age of 50 has increased sharply with important implications for treatment programmes in low- and middle-income countries that will need to focus on integrated health and social services to cater for the changing care needs of PLHIV as they age (Autenrieth et al., 2018).

The 69% decline in global AIDS-related deaths with ever widening access to effective ART obscures the harsh reality that over 40 million people are thought to have died since HIV type 1 crossed the species barrier from chimpanzees and became pandemic. In contrast, some 15 million people are estimated to have died with COVID-19, albeit over a much shorter time-frame.

The annual numbers are aggregate figures. When looked at by region, it is clear that the heaviest burden of HIV disease and AIDS remains in sub-Saharan Africa, still the home of two-thirds of all PLHIV. Within sub-Saharan Africa, eastern and southern Africa is the epicentre of continued transmission. This region has made the most impressive gains in HIV treatment, with ART coverage second only to Western Europe and North America. However, services are not equally taken up with significant gender gaps: heterosexual men particularly those aged 35–49 represent the largest unaddressed gap in HIV services currently (Cornell et al., 2021).

Stratification by region, gender, age or vulnerability identifies two critical issues for HIV prevention to address and highlight the need for countries to know their epidemic, and know their response:

- *Vulnerability of young women in sub-Saharan Africa*: globally every week in 2022, 4,000 young women aged 15–24 years became infected with HIV; around 80% occurred in sub-Saharan Africa. Here, six in seven new infections among adolescents aged 15–19 years are among girls; girls and young women aged 15–24 years are three times more likely to be living with HIV than young men of the same age; women and girls accounted for nearly two-thirds of all new infections in sub-Saharan Africa.
- *Importance of key populations in maintaining HIV transmission*: in 2021, key populations (female sex workers and their clients; gay men and other men who have sex with men; people who inject drugs; transgender people) and their sexual partners accounted for 70% of HIV infections globally: 94% of new infections outside sub-Saharan Africa are in key populations, compared with just over half in sub-Saharan Africa. The risk of acquiring HIV is 35 times higher in PWID; 30 times higher for FSW that adult women; 28 times higher for men who have sex with men than adult heterosexual men; and 14 times higher for TG women than adult women (Joint United Nations Programme on HIV/AIDS (UNAIDS), 2022).

If HIV transmission is to be further contained, then globally combination prevention will need a more intense focus on key populations: countries need to better know their epidemic and their response to optimally allocate resources to their specific key populations. In sub-Saharan Africa, targeted interventions are needed to reduce the risks and vulnerability of young and adolescent women and to better address the structural barriers to accessing and using HIV prevention services.

Treatment programmes need to continue to drive up ART coverage in all juris-dictions; to identify the gaps in use of HIV services and structural barriers limit-ing access to ART; define important drops in the cascade of care and address the likely reasons for these falls to increase retention in care, and cope with an ageing population of PLHIV. Maintaining the survival benefit for the individual and at the population level needs a continued focus on providing optimal care and viral suppression.

How an effective response to the AIDS epidemic helped invent global health

One significant consequence of the evolving response to HIV/AIDS has been to disrupt the traditional boundaries between public health and primary healthcare (PHC) and clinical medicine and hospital-based service delivery; and especially the divide between disease prevention and care and treatment. An exceptional response to AIDS has driven scientific advances that have made HIV simple to diagnose accurately, made highly effective ART easy to use and introduced game-changing biomedical prevention. New financing mechanisms have been created to close the treatment gap and to support combination prevention. Pro-grammatic successes make achieving the SDG HIV/AIDS targets feasible for most countries.

AIDS activists highlighted the primacy of human rights in the response, including the rights to treatment and care and non-discrimination, and helped reshape cultural attitudes and social behaviours. International solidarity at the UN between public health officials, funders, politicians and community leaders has been instrumental in setting global health policy and accorded HIV/AIDS a prominent place in the millennium development goals (MDGs) then the SDGs. It has upended conventional wisdom around public health in the global south, moving on from the old, traditional approaches embodied in what was called international health to the new and distinct construct called global health.

Global health is distinct for several reasons, all of which have emerged from the activities and actions developed to respond so successfully to HIV/AIDS:

- It recognises the essential supranational character of disease and effective interventions including legislation.
- It focusses on deeper knowledge of the burden of disease, key health dis-parities and the social determinants of health to develop strategies for their control or reduction.
- It recognises the centrality of community for equitable access and person-centred care.
- It is based on ethical and moral values and recognises that equity and rights are central to the larger goals preventing and treating disease, and universal health coverage.

It can be argued that without the AIDS epidemic there would be no global health movement as we know it today; AIDS invented global health (Brandt, 2013).

Programme disruptions and stresses with the SARS-CoV-2/ COVID-19 pandemic

On 30 January 2020, WHO declared the SARSCoV2/COVID-19 outbreak a Public Health Emergency of International Concern (PHEIC). With this, important global recommendations were made to deal with the sudden challenges posed by the emerging pandemic: to support countries with weaker health systems; accelerate the development of vaccines, therapeutics and diagnostics; review preparedness plans; identify gaps and evaluate the resources needed to identify, isolate and care for sick COVID-19 patients; and prevent transmission. In particular, the PHEIC required enhanced surveillance by WHO member states and to report the outbreak and evolution of disease to WHO as stipulated by the International Health Regulations (IHR) (Merianos & Peiris, 2005). Rapid progress has been made in SARSCoV2 diagnostics, disease management and vaccine development; COVAX (the COVID-19 Vaccines Global Access) has delivered 2 billion vaccine doses to 146 countries and made attempts to establish more equity and diversification of vaccine and diagnostic production.

It is clear that over a short time period the pandemic has exposed weaknesses in the health systems of low- and middle-income countries. The impact of the rapid shift in focus to COVID-19 on routine health services and disease control programmes for tuberculosis, malaria and HIV/AIDS have been dramatic. Health services have been disrupted, and the diversion of already limited resources and staff away from these routine services and control programmes is threatening to reverse some of the gains made towards achieving global disease control targets. Movement restrictions and lock-downs have limited the ability of patients to access HIV testing services or to attend clinic for review and ART refills (Izudi et al., 2022).

The exceptionalism and special focus on HIV/AIDS that had ensured that health services rolled out and delivered effective ART and combination prevention to all in need was significantly disrupted and overtaken by the new pandemic. WHO's recommendations for a public health approach for HIV/ AIDS programmes were predicated on having available the necessary human resources, diagnostics and medicines; it was not designed to be robust to *force majeure* and the sudden reprioritisation away from HIV/AIDS services.

With limited country-level data, the impact of COVID-19 disease is yet to be fully quantified. Globally the number of people on ART grew more slowly in 2021 than it has in over a decade (Joint United Nations Programme on HIV/ AIDS (UNAIDS), 2022). In adults living with HIV in South Africa and using public sector healthcare, COVID-19 mortality is strongly associated with suboptimal HIV control: it remains a public health priority to ensure PLHIV are on suppressive ART and are fully vaccinated against SARSCoV2 (Kassanjee et al., 2023). Income inequality is globally associated with less effective pandemic responses: more unequal countries show higher AIDS mortality and COVID-19 excess mortality (Ataguba et al., 2023).

At the population level, there have already been millions of excess deaths directly and indirectly related to COVID-19 and more will follow, as healthcare systems slowly return to normal, and the backlog of care is dealt with. The full impact will be modelled rather than counted because of the weakness of civil registration, vital statistics and data collection in resource-poor countries: this impedes efforts to convince donors and governments of the need to invest more resources to revamp health services and for pandemic preparedness (Chanda-Kapata et al., 2022).

On 5 May 2023, WHO DG Tedros Adhanom Ghebreyesus accepted advice from his staff to end the COVID-19 PHEIC, saying that it was time for countries to transition from emergency mode to managing COVID-19 alongside other infectious diseases. WHO will shift its focus towards the management of the disease as an established and ongoing health issue, integrated into routine health programmes. Health services in low- and middle-income countries are expected quickly to recover with resources (human and financial) re-prioritised back into disease-specific control programmes including HIV/AIDS.

The decision to end the emergency after less than 30 months was welcomed by many global health leaders who considered that no disease should be in a chronic state of emergency that goes on for years as this can dilute the power of calling an emergency in the first place (Zarocostas, 2023). This contrasts with the prolonged state of emergency that characterises messaging around the HIV/AIDS epidemic, and that was the driver for civil society and PLHIV to demand an exceptional response initially in the United States and then globally (Smith & Whiteside, 2010).

Challenges with sustaining and growing the finances needed to end AIDS

Fast-tracking the response, getting to zero new infections and accelerating action towards the end of AIDS by 2030 requires that the HIV response will receive additional financing that is sustained into the future. Prevention services need additional resources to better target key populations and young vulnerable women. In the absence of a cure, to keep pace with new patients starting ART, the ever-rising number who are alive but need continued ART for life and the growing demand for biomedical prevention, budgets to procure ARVs will need to increase year-on-year. Furthermore, an ageing population of PLHIV will need access to a wider, more costly range of health and social services.

For over a decade the data unfortunately shows that there has been very little additional financing. The Kaiser Foundation and UNAIDS have tracked donor

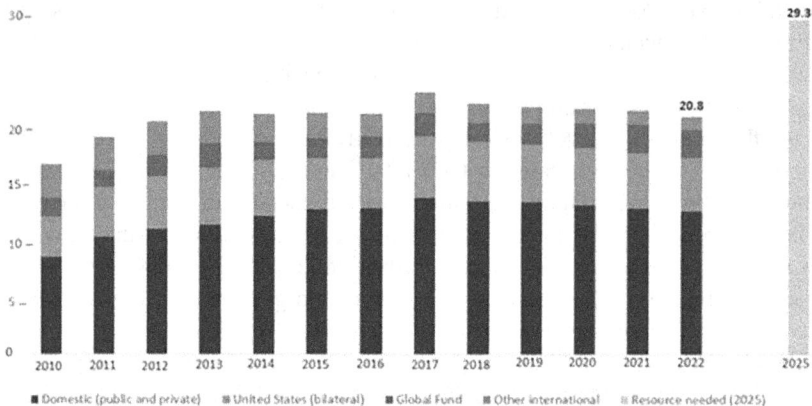

Figure 5.1 Global financing for AIDS control from domestic and international sources

government funding for HIV, assessing both bilateral disbursements and multi-lateral contributions over the MDG era. Resources available for HIV in low- and middle-income countries have more or less flat-lined since 2008, and therefore been declining in real terms, at a time when they need to increase to accommodate wider use of ART and ARVs for biomedical prevention. Around 40% of the resource envelope for AIDS programming was bilateral, with several governments providing a greater share of funding than others and relative to their GDP: this includes the United States, the United Kingdom, Norway and Denmark (Kates et al., 2014).

International development assistance for HIV/AIDS has continued to flat-line as the SDGs have replaced the MDGs. Domestic public funding and inputs from the private sector have been maintained and marginally increased covering around 60% of AIDS programme financing. For 2021, UNAIDS reported that while US$21.4 billion was available for the AIDS response in low- and middle-income countries, this was far short of the estimated annual requirements, estimated for 2025, of US$ 29 billion needed to keep on track to end AIDS by 2030. Coupled with the major disruptions caused by SARSCoV2/COVID-19 and the stresses of returning quickly to pre-pandemic services, it seems that progress towards ending AIDS is slowing and may be in imminent danger (Joint United Nations Programme on HIV/AIDS (UNAIDS), 2022) (Figure 5.1).

The Global Fund and PEPFAR were established following the UN Declaration of Commitment on HIV/AIDS to provide funds to support an exceptional global response to closing the treatment gap (United Nations (UN), 2001). Subsequent UN General Assembly political declarations on HIV and AIDS have committed to ambitious new goals and targets, and most recently in 2021 pledged to end inequalities and get on track to end AIDS by 2030 (United Nations (UN),

2021). But no new funding mechanisms nor additional funds for HIV/AIDS programmes have emerged.

Worryingly, rather than ramping up their global AIDS funding, PEPFAR may be slackening off its investment (Honermann et al., 2023). The most recent Global Fund replenishment round asked for at least US $18 billion to finance its activities for 2023–2025: in the event it raised just US $14.25 billion (Burki, 2022). Collectively these global funding mechanisms seem unlikely to be able to cover the growing budget shortfalls.

Some low- and middle-income countries could mobilise additional domestic resources but the majority will at best maintain existing financing (Haakenstad et al., 2019). The burden of disease in the global south is rapidly changing, as widely anticipated by the epidemiological transition model, and non-communicable diseases (NCDs) are emerging as the new public health priorities for action. Despite this, limited funding has been directed to manage and control NCDs (Santosa et al., 2014). In this environment, it seems unlikely that further exceptional AIDS funding will be forthcoming from domestic budgets sources to cover shortfalls or even sustain current programme funding.

What is to be done? Preparing for endemic HIV and the end of AIDS

Globally, the number of new HIV infections has been steadily decreasing since the mid-late 1990s when they peaked. Although no country has yet declared it has got to zero new infections, all the indications are that the HIV epidemic is now over, except in some key populations and especially vulnerable groups, and that HIV is endemic. However, without further scaling up of combination prevention HIV incidence is unlikely to fall to zero or become endemic in vulnerable and key populations by 2030 or sometime soon after.

In contrast, with high treatment coverage, AIDS deaths have continuing steadily to decrease from their peak in the early 2000s as ART roll out started to go to scale. If progress is maintained, many countries will be on track to end AIDS as a public health problem by 2030 (Figure 5.2).

Even if HIV is eliminated as a public health threat and AIDS is ended by 2030, there can be no end game: HIV prevention cannot suddenly cease, nor can treatment stop in 2031. Without a cure, ART has to be given for life: if stopped, viral load will rise, individuals will become capable of onward HIV transmission, develop AIDS and then die prematurely. Prevention has to continue for as long as people are on ART; if it stops or is dramatically wound down, a second HIV epidemic is inevitable. Clarion calls to end AIDS by 2030 disguise the imperative for sustained programming and continued funding for the foreseeable future (Assefa & Gilks, 2020).

What then needs to be done to sustain, let alone grow, the resource envelope for the foreseeable future? Perhaps the time is right now to move away from

Number of AIDS-related deaths and new HIV infections globally, 1990-2022

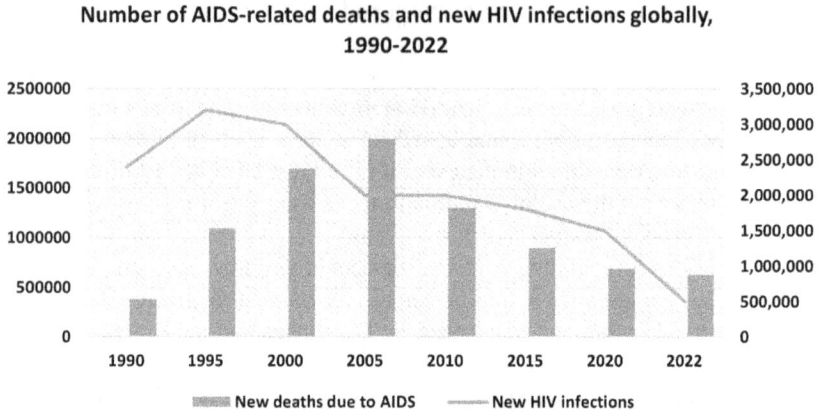

Figure 5.2 Number of new HIV infections and AIDS deaths from 1990 to 2022

target-driven campaigning, recognising the huge impact this had to kick-start ART scale-up and then sustain a consolidated response covering prevention, testing, treatment, service delivery and monitoring.

- It seems sensible to acknowledge that HIV/AIDS is now well beyond the global public health emergency it once was, that demanded an exceptional response and significant earmarked funding to cope equitably with the epidemic in the global south.
- Language around the HIV epidemic should be revised in favour of endemic HIV, particularly when most countries are in the endemic phase. This will help drive the fact that come what may in 2030, while the endemic phase lasts, prevention has to be continued long-term.
- Language around the end of AIDS may better emphasise that HIV infection is a chronic disease needing lifelong ART, with no possibility to end it (Deeks et al., 2013).
- Calls for one more thrust to end AIDS should be tempered. It seems not to have worked for a long time, as earmarked AIDS funding has flat-lined since 2008 and shows no sign of growing. What happens in the run-up to 2030 if the call for action is ignored as it may well be?
- Suggesting that insufficient investment has put the global response in danger as UNAIDS has done risks becoming counter-productive even as the world looks to ending AIDS by 2030 (Joint United Nations Programme on HIV/ AIDS (UNAIDS), 2022).
- The burden of disease in low- and middle-income countries is fast shifting to the NCDs, as are priorities for disease control and funding. More resources are needed for strengthened health services to match the burden of disease.

- Playing to one's strengths is more productive. So much has been achieved from a very low base to end AIDS deaths and turn the epidemic into the endemic; given the nature of HIV and the lack of a vaccine or cure the response has to be sustained medium and long-term.

UNAIDS more recently has made it clear that there is a path to end AIDS: HIV responses succeed when they are anchored in strong political leadership; countries that put people and communities first in policy and practice are leading the world on the journey to end AIDS by 2030. But the call remains for further sustained funding for vertical programming (Joint UNAIDS Programme on HIV/AIDS (UNAIDS), 2023).

While much is AIDS programme specific, some clearly links to other disease control programmes which have different funding streams. WHO has identified NCD actions and services to be prioritised and integrated into HIV service packages. Countries are already moving on this, for example, Eswatini and South Africa have demonstrated person-centred models for HIV and NCD integration through decentralised drug distribution (Goldstein, Ford, et al., 2023).

TB/HIV coinfection is common and usually managed by TB control programmes; A Kenyan study noted that systematic HIV testing is needed to ensure outcome is optimised (Ngari et al., 2023). Tuberculosis preventive therapy substantially reduces the risks of PLHIV developing active disease; a national campaign substantially increased IPT use in Uganda (Musaazi et al., 2023). PMCTC services can be integrated within MCH services, with them assuming responsibility for driving infant HIV infection to zero.

Calls for resources to support HIV/AIDS activities do not have to come from or be managed by AIDS programmes. They can be made by other disease control programmes, especially when they are more likely to be listened to and acted on, as priorities change and shift to NCDs for example, or child survival. They can be jointly made, as the US Agency for International Development has suggested, to support the integration of stand-alone HIV programming with PHC platforms with strategic funding flexibly provided by international assistance from donor governments (Goldstein et al., 2023).

Better still they could be made under the banner of health systems strengthening (HSS): the Global Fund has a specific HSS focus and many bilateral donors are keen to fund it as part of international development assistance (Waife et al., 2019). Indeed, an HSS approach can address some perverse consequences and potential outcomes of ending AIDS. Budget holders may be tempted to reduce activities and cut budgets without recognising the ongoing need to have an experienced and skilled workforce to deliver combination prevention and effective ART. Some clinicians are already wondering what happens to the HIV testing workforce when the epidemic ends (Green, 2022).

Looking to the future, HIV/AIDS services will need to be continued for as long as HIV is endemic and PLHIV are on ART. A note of realism must now start to be given, that we are in it for the long haul to sustain the impressive gains already made and that ending AIDS cannot mean skilled workforces are disbanded and services come to an end. Funding to support health systems rather than vertical disease control programmes that are often in competition with each other in fragmented health services may be a better way to support person-centred care and integrated service delivery at the primary care and district levels. It may also be the best way to support actions under SDG 3, ensuring healthy lives and promote well-being for all at all ages, and for delivering on the NCD agenda and moving towards UHC.

These issues are explored further in the next two sections of the book.

Section 2

A public health approach for NCD control in the global south

6 Chronic non-communicable diseases as a global public health challenge

The epidemiological transition from malnutrition and infection to chronic disease

Over centuries, there have been profound changes in fertility, life expectancy, mortality and causes of death across almost all societies. These transitions, linked with improved food security, wealth, socio-economic development and innovations in public health and medicine have had different impacts on population growth and fertility rates and have not happened in a uniform fashion at country level. Nevertheless, such transitions can account for the replacement of infectious diseases by chronic diseases over time as a result of improved healthcare and disease prevention.

In 1971, Dr Abdel Omran proposed a theory of epidemiological transition (ET) linking patterns of health and disease with demographic, economic and sociological determinants that were able to describe changing population patterns in terms of fertility, diet and nutrition, life expectancy, mortality and leading causes of death. He divided the transition of mortality into three phases; in 1998 he updated this to a five-stage construct (Omran, 1998):

1 The age of pestilence and famine: high mortality from infectious diseases, malnutrition and famine precluding population growth; life expectancy was short, between 20 and 40 years.
2 The age of receding pandemics: mortality progressively declines as epidemics decrease in frequency, allowing sustained population growth; life expectancy increases from 30 to 50 years; population growth is sustained and begins to be exponential.
3 The age of degenerative and man-made diseases: mortality continues to decline and is increasingly related to degenerative diseases, cardiovascular disease (CVD), cancer, violence and substance use; life expectancy exceeds 50 years, fertility governs population growth.
4 The age of declining CVD mortality, ageing and emerging diseases: CVD diminishes as a cause of mortality due to changes in culture, lifestyle, diet and

DOI: 10.4324/9781003505693-9

advances in medicine; the birth rate levels off although emerging diseases can become significant causes of mortality
5 The age of aspired quality of life with persistent inequalities: birth rate declines as lifespan extends, leading to an age-balanced population; genetic predisposition with socio-economic, ethnic and gender inequalities continue to impact mortality and fertility.

Rapid declines in mortality rates and overall improvement in health was particularly dramatic in the second half of the 20th century, when the theory of ET emerged. Yet despite huge overall global improvements in health, many low- and middle-income countries have not shared in the gains or have fallen further behind high-income countries. Originally framed from the perspective of industrialised countries, much of the research and writings on ET theory now consider low- and middle-income countries that are all experiencing the transition to chronic diseases, albeit at different levels of progress in terms of time, pace of change and drivers of the transition.

The observed demographic and economic changes have not always followed the pathways described in the original ET construct, with partial concordance between established theory and empirical evidence, especially around mortality rates. In the 1990s the World Bank first started to work on disease control priorities (DCP-1) in developing countries, an attempt to assess systematically value for money, using cost-effectiveness analysis of interventions that would address the major sources of disease burden in low- and middle-income countries. It introduced the concept of a protracted ET involving a dual burden of chronic non-communicable diseases (NCDs) combined with the lingering problems of infectious disease (Jamison & Mosley, 1991). Income inequality is one driver yet improvements in health can arise without rapidly growing incomes. Correct policies promoting the best health interventions can greatly reduce mortality, one reason why health policy development has figured so prominently in the chronic NCDs response.

It has also been suggested, that classic ET theory rather neglected the social determinants of health (SDH) and more contemporary issues like climate change (Santosa et al., 2014). The idea that social factors were an important determinant of disease outcome grew from a study of British civil servants, government office workers in Whitehall, that showed the importance of social class in determining health inequalities and disease susceptibility: the lower the social class, the higher the mortality rate. In the United Kingdom, the term inequalities has traditionally been used to describe the differences in health between groups defined on the basis of class and socio-economic conditions; in other jurisdictions, these are referred to as health inequities (Marmot et al., 1991).

Beyond a framework to describe inequality and social disadvantage as a major determinant of health gaps in society, in the spirit of social justice the Commission on Social Determinants of Health was set up by WHO in 2005 to marshal evidence on what can be done to promote health equity and to foster a global movement to achieve it. The commission had three overarching recommendations: to improve daily living conditions; to tackle the inequitable distribution of power, money and resources; and to measure and understand the problem and assess the impact of specific actions (WHO Commission on Social Determinants of Health, 2008).

Whatever theoretical framework or body of research is used, and actions proposed to try to address the drivers, the ET from malnutrition and infection to other morbid conditions, particularly chronic diseases that are not directly transmissible from one person to another, has resulted in significant changes in the burden of disease in the global south. The shift to chronic diseases has been an increasing focus of attention of the UN, multilateral organisations like WHO, development agencies and of the global health movement.

Highlighting the global importance of chronic non-communicable diseases and the need for action

An appreciation of the rising burden of chronic diseases in low- and middle-income countries and the changing global burden of disease (GBD) has been developing for over 50 years. It started with ET theory in 1971, predominantly focussing on high-income settings. The social determinants of health studies highlighted the importance of social factors. In the 1990s, the GBD study sponsored by WHO and the World Bank started to assemble data sets comprehensive enough to describe the world's health and to set priorities for health services and research. The fifth and final round quantified the burdens of 483 sequelae of 109 major causes of death and disability disaggregated by eight geographical regions and ten age-sex groups, with projections to the year 2020 (Murray & Lopez, 1996).

In 2001, the World Bank and the US National Institutes of Health started a new project with the DCP team to identify policy changes and intervention strategies for the major health problems of low- and middle-income countries across a broad range of diseases and conditions. It continued to state the importance of communicable diseases and nutrition and illness and mortality in children; it drew attention to the emergence of chronic NCDs. For prevention and treatment programmes to work across these different disease groups, policymakers need the best possible research and analysis to ensure their health investments save as many lives as possible.

The DCP project focussed strongly on the assessment of cost-effectiveness of health-improving interventions for the conditions responsible for the greatest burden of disease. Cost-effectiveness data indicate what a reasonably well-functioning health system can achieve. They need to be supplemented with evidence and guidance on how health systems can be strengthened to provide interventions effectively, efficiently and equitably. Increasing the flow of resources to health, drawing on both donor support and national spending is essential to implement priority interventions. It culminated in the second edition, known as DCP-2 (Laxminarayan et al., 2006).

Building on the initial GBD studies, WHO's World Health Report 2002 "Reducing risks, promoting healthy life" drew attention to the importance of chronic NCDs, the need to reduce their risk profiles and to focus on their prevention. It discussed a disease risk transition, similar to the demographic transition (World Health Organization (WHO), 2002). The Lancet with WHO and other partners then brought together leading experts and researchers working in chronic diseases and formed the Chronic Diseases Action Group to strengthen the evidence for prevention by publishing three Series of papers.

The first Series, "The neglected epidemic of chronic disease" was published in 2005 in association with a powerful WHO report, "Chronic disease prevention: a vital investment" (World Health Organization (WHO), 2005a). It highlighted the huge burden of chronic diseases in low- and low-middle-income countries: while 35 million people were projected to die in 2005 from heart disease, stroke, cancer and other chronic diseases, only 20% were in high-income settings with 80% in the global south. It appropriately called this a neglected epidemic, proposed a goal of reducing death rates by an additional 2% annually in order to avert 36 million deaths by 2015, and urged coordinated political and stepwise health-system action to reduce the impact of the epidemic of chronic diseases (Strong et al., 2005).

The second Lancet Series "Chronic diseases: the case for global action" was published two years later (Horton, 2007). Three cost-effective interventions, tobacco control, salt reduction and combined drug treatment for people at high absolute risk of CVD could avert over 30 million deaths over a ten-year period at an annual cost of approximately US$ 6 billion. This was noted to be about half the cost of providing medicines for ART (Gazianoet al., 2007). It ended with a call for action from all stakeholders, especially development agencies, donor countries and private foundations which continued to neglect the prevention of chronic disease despite the robust scientific basis for action (Beaglehole et al., 2007).

The third and final Lancet Series "Chronic diseases as a development issue" followed three years later (Beaglehole & Horton, 2010). It started from the premise that our collective failure to address the chronic disease pandemic was a political rather than technical failure, given that proven cost-effective interventions were available. Advancing chronic disease prevention required re-framing development discussions to emphasise the underlying social determinants of disease and the inter-relationship between chronic disease, poverty and development. Resources needed to be mobilised through an inclusive approach; and distributed more equitably on the basis of avoidable mortality rather than primarily on fashionable diseases like HIV/AIDS (Geneau et al., 2010).

A package of measures to tackle unhealthy diets, physical inactivity and obesity could deliver substantial health gains at a cost ranging from US$ 1.3 to US$ 4.5 per person, with very favourable cost-effectiveness ratios (Cecchini et al., 2010). While health system strengthening (HSS) was receiving increasing attention, the focus was on infectious diseases and MNCH services. It was equally important for patients at risk of or experiencing chronic diseases: policymakers and health practitioners were urged not to treat chronic diseases as an after-thought (Samb et al., 2010).

Despite all this effort by academics and public health practitioners there was limited recognition of the importance of chronic diseases globally, and the pressing need to take action. In contrast to communicable diseases like HIV/AIDS, TB and malaria, chronic diseases did not figure significantly in the Millennium Development Goals for 2015, despite their strong focus on health; and even though the overall development goals of poverty reduction, health equity, economic stability and human security were at risk without concerted action to combat the neglected epidemic of chronic diseases.

In stark contrast to AIDS, there was limited civil society activism for any of the priority chronic diseases, there were no vocal country champions, no special funding mechanism were being proposed and inadequate earmarked funds were being provided to combat the neglected epidemic of chronic diseases in the global south.

There was a pivot globally in the framing of chronic diseases to rebrand them as NCDs to better distinguish them from the fashionable communicable diseases with special funding mechanisms. The Lancet established an NCD action group, an informal collaboration of academics, practitioners and civil society organisations; and linked with the NCD alliance, four key international non-government organisations in cancer, lung disease, diabetes and heart disease.

The failure to create a sustained global movement was now called the NCD crisis and priority actions in leadership, prevention, treatment, international cooperation and monitoring and accountability were identified to address this (Beaglehole, Bonita, Horton, et al., 2011). The major NCD groups – diabetes, cancer, CVDs and chronic respiratory diseases – had shared risk factors in tobacco use, harmful use of alcohol, unhealthy diets and physical inactivity.

The NCD action group and NCD alliance paper was timed to appear just before the UN convened the first high-level meeting (HLM) on NCDs, seen as an unprecedented opportunity to stimulate a coordinated international response to NCDs that would be commensurate with their health impacts and economic burdens (United Nations (UN), 2011). Parallels were drawn with the 2001 UNGASS special session on HIV/AIDS which had recognised that dealing with the epidemic was central to the development agenda.

A global multisectoral response was required to impact the NCD crisis; the efficient use of existing resources and new innovative financing methods were needed, rather than setting up a new global fund. Long-term success in implementing the commitments to action were acknowledged to be dependent on inspired and committed national and international leadership (Beaglehole et al., 2011).

Following the 2011 HLM for NCDs, there was an urgent need for policies and strategies that prevent NCDs by reducing their major risk factors with a broader notion of preventability than detecting causes that increase disease risk in individuals. Ten effective approaches were highlighted ranging from tobacco and alcohol control, dietary interventions, clean fuels for cooking, vaccination and screening and treatment of NCDs in primary care. Policies and actions to change NCD risk factors need political support and policy and administrative institutions that can initiate, evaluate and as necessary redirect them. Many actions can prevent multiple NCDs and can have large benefits on the health of populations as well as individuals (Ezzati & Riboli, 2012).

In 2013, WHO produced a global action plan (GAP) for the prevention and control of NCDs that provided member states, international partners and WHO with a road map and menu of policy options which if implemented could result in a 25% relative reduction in premature mortality from NCDs by 2025. The vision was for a world free of the avoidable burden of NCDs; the goal was to reduce preventable and avoidable morbidity, mortality and disability due to NCDs by multisectoral collaboration at national, regional and global levels so that populations reach the highest attainable standards of health and productivity at every age and so those diseases are no longer a barrier to well-being or socio-economic development.

The plan relied on overarching principles including a human rights and equity-based approach, national multisectoral action, international cooperation and solidarity, a life course approach, empowerment of peoples and communities, evidence-based strategies, universal health coverage (UHC) and the management of conflicts of interest where public health action may be compromised by vested interests (Table 6.1). It had six objectives and a suite of voluntary global targets that ranged from reducing population salt intake, increasing physical activity and mortality reduction: some were behavioural; others were clinical (World Health Organization (WHO), 2013).

In the same year, The Lancet Commission on Investing in Health revisited the case for investment in health and developed a new investment framework to achieve dramatic health gains by 2035. It heavily drew on the DCP project and had four key messages, each of which contained opportunities for action by national governments of low- and middle-income countries and by the international community. There is an enormous payoff from investing in health and a strong case for allocating a higher proportion of development aid to health.

A grand convergence is possible with the ever-improving technical capacity to reduce infectious, child and maternal mortality rates significantly across the global south. Fiscal policies are a powerful and underutilised lever for curbing chronic NCDs and injuries. Pro-poor pathways and progressive universalism are efficient ways to achieve health and financial protection and a pathway to UHC. The commission was looking beyond the chronic NCD agenda towards ways to achieve UHC (Jamison et al., 2013).

Table 6.1 The six objectives in the WHO Global Action Plan (GAP) for the prevention and control of non-communicable diseases 2013–2020

	Global action plan 2013 objectives
Objective 1	To raise priority accorded to the prevention and control of NCDs in global, regional and national agendas and internationally agreed development goals, through strengthened international cooperation and advocacy
Objective 2	To strengthen national capacity, leadership, governance, multisectoral action and partnerships to accelerate country responses for the prevention and control of NCDs
Objective 3	To reduce modifiable risk factors for NCDs and the underlying social determinants through the creation of health-promoting environments
Objective 4	To strengthen and orient health systems to address the prevention and control of NCDs and the underlying social determinants through people-centred primary health care and universal health coverage
Objective 5	To promote and support national capacity for high-quality research and development for the prevention and control of NCDs
Objective 6	To monitor the trends and determinants on NCDs and evaluate progress in their prevention and control

The complex chronic non-communicable disease construct

Despite the initial high-level discussion at the UN, at WHO and in leading academic journals on the importance of epidemic chronic diseases as a development issue with a vital case for investment and clear priorities for action, there was a crisis in the failure to create a sustained global movement for NCD prevention and control and to generate momentum for actions and impact at country level. Some of this may have been due to confusion about what exactly the chronic NCDs are and the heterogenous domains for risk reduction they present: much is in the construct.

Diseases are named and grouped together in bewildering and sometimes contradictory ways. Some names have broad recognition and meaning that is understood by health practitioners, global health experts, consumers and the lay public alike; other names and labels are more technical or medical with restricted use and limited recognition outside clinical or public health circles. There is no common approach, agreed taxonomy or set of rules to follow when naming a new disease. Existing names have emerged over time in a whole variety of ways: names and meanings have also changed over time as medical science has advanced, and disease aetiology is better understood.

In biblical times, illnesses like plague, leprosy and the pox and processes like famine and maternal mortality were understood and widely feared; contagions like plague or leprosy were stigmatising and have remained so today. Some names, like diabetes, measles, malnutrition or cholera are in common parlance and widely used; others like kwashiorkor or kuru have more restricted usage but deep community meaning. Names can be derived from organs and disease processes: breast cancer; duodenal ulcer; pneumonia. They can be eponymous like Cushing's disease, named after their discoverer; an acronym like SARS or AIDS; or be from a place associated with the disease, like Ebola or Spanish flu, although this practice is now frowned upon. Obesity is now widely regarded as a disease or illness, as well as being a risk factor for several NCDs.

Correctly diagnosing disease is the fundamental axis of clinical practice for both patient and health practitioner: it requires the disease to have an identity and name; it is the entry point for treatment and for establishing prognosis. At the population level, the importance of accurate and consistent use of a disease name is often undervalued and underappreciated, despite the fact that it is core for epidemiology; and fundamental for measuring and understanding disease to inform prevention, treatment and optimal resource allocation. To be useful, measurement must be reliable, allow valid comparisons over place and time and enable coherent summarisation of large volumes of data. A globally accepted classification of disease is essential for this.

The International Classification of Diseases (ICD) has long been the main basis for comparability of statistics on causes of morbidity and mortality between places and over time: it is in its eleventh iteration, ICD-11 (Harrison et al., 2021). It has approximately 80,000 entries complemented by 40,000 synonyms, each characterising a disease, syndrome or health-related phenomenon. A specific diagnosis is usually represented by a single code with mechanisms to allow codes to be clustered for analysis or reporting.

ICD-coded data have for many years been the basis of international and national statistics on cause-specific mortality. As regards the major NCDs: CVD has ICD-10 codes I00–I99; diabetes IC-10 codes E10–14; chronic respiratory diseases ICD-10 codes J40–J47 and diseases of the digestive system ICD-10 codes K00–K93. The mortality data along with ICD-coded morbidity data have been crucial inputs to estimates of burden of disease and injury at a global and local level and to identify significant changes in single disease incidence.

The original GBD study has been expanded to become the Global Burden of Diseases Injuries and Risk Factors Study. In an era of shifting global agendas and an expanded emphasis on NCDs and injuries along with communicable diseases, sound evidence on trends by cause at national level is essential. It provides a systematic assessment of data on incidence, prevalence and mortality for a mutually exhaustive list of diseases and injuries. The initial GBD studies had 483 sequelae of 109 major causes of death; the 2019 GBD study now estimates incidence, prevalence, mortality and disability-adjusted life years due to

369 major diseases and injuries (Vos et al., 2020). It is a much simpler classification to use than the ICD.

Diseases are grouped together in a wide variety of ways, according to system, process, aetiology, social practice, socio-economic status or mode of transmission: many overlap and a specific disease can be categorised into different groups. There are diseases common to one organ or system, like cardiovascular or respiratory disease. Diseases can be grouped by pathological or causative process: cancer, infarct, infection, organ failure, genetic, accident, adverse drug reaction, injury or trauma. They can be classified by place: community-acquired; nosocomial; by mode of transmission: water-wash and water-borne, airborne aerosol, sexually transmitted or blood-borne; by social and economic factors: addiction, alcohol, diet and exercise, lifestyle, disease of poverty or affluence, substance use. Some are grouped around a common theme: acute, chronic, non-communicable, neglected tropical, vaccine-preventable and so on. Several groupings around organ system or process are chapter headers in the ICD; or are a cause in the GBD. They lead to individual diseases.

The initial GBD studies erected a tripartite high-level classification system for disease and injury creating three major groups for ease of reporting and analysis: communicable, maternal, perinatal and nutritional conditions; NCDs; and injuries (Murray & Lopez, 1996). The ICD has a variable-axis classification with five major groupings: epidemic disease; constitutional or general diseases; local diseases arranged by site; developmental diseases; and injuries. It does not have a specific header or entry for either chronic diseases or NCDs; they are invisible at the macro level. Particular diseases need to be individually identified and then aggregated for any analysis of NCD trends. Neither chronic disease nor NCDs figure in any of the major textbooks of medicine.

Names and labels are important. The public are much more likely to invest in and support campaigns if they are aware of the disease: breast cancer awareness, world AIDS day or world immunisation week. Politicians will be more willing to develop policy and invest in a control programme if it is valued domestically and recognisable as worthwhile; and allocate development assistance to a problem discussed by the UN and clearly identified as a priority for action. Chronic diseases that are not directly transmissible from person to person was never a construct understood by voters or politicians. Grouping disparate diseases under the NCD banner does not translate into recognisable problems like diabetes, heart disease or cancer except for people familiar with health: planners and policymakers, public health experts and global health academics who understand the agenda.

Highlighting that the NCDs are complex to prevent or manage, or what the NCDs are not is hardly best practice in branding and communication. It can be confusing when several priority cancers in the global south result from chronic viral infection and are thus vaccine-preventable: cervical cancer and oncogenic strains of human papilloma virus; hepatocellular cancer and chronic hepatitis B virus infection; nasopharyngeal and mouth cancers and Epstein-Barr virus. It has however clearly distinguished the NCDs from HIV/AIDS, TB and malaria, the fashionable communicable disease control priorities in the global south which have received special attention and generous funding.

In a similar fashion, a set of communicable diseases largely restricted to the tropics have been branded together as the neglected tropical diseases (NTDs) to highlight the limited attention and funding they receive in comparison to the big three infections with specific funding channels in the global fund; and for HIV/ AIDS an exceptional global response.

The communicable vs non-communicable binary is problematic because it encourages planners and policymakers to view HIV/AIDS and NCDs as separate and very different health challenges. This false dichotomy obscures the core fact that HIV/AIDS and the individual NCDs like diabetes or CVD are complex to prevent, with a challenging mix of structural, lifestyle, behavioural and biomedical interventions needed at individual and population level. There are important lessons from successful HIV/AIDS control programmes that are directly relevant to NCD control because of the similarities in disease processes and health service responses that are irrespective of being transmissible or not.

Despite combination prevention, many end up with disease that needs to be effectively diagnosed and managed. The other false dichotomy is the tension in public health action between prevention or treatment, when in fact it has to be both; individuals or communities with a preventable disease will need some form of care and treatment when prevention has not worked. There are important similarities with HIV/AIDS and NCD treatment and care: both are seemingly complex to treat at the primary care level and will often need specialist management and hospital care.

A crucial and rarely acknowledged further similarity is that they cannot be cured: following screening and diagnosis, treatment is lifelong and without an obvious end-point. With a public health approach to ART making the end of AIDS by 2030 achievable in most of the global south, this should inspire NCD programme managers to focus on common programmatic challenges in delivering long-term care support and treatment for NCDs and HIV/AIDS and to translate the successes achieved in one communicable disease programme across the divide to NCDs.

If there were a better name to encompass the cumbersome NCD construct with its principal diseases and their shared risk factors to make it more understandable and accessible to multiple stakeholders then it would surely have emerged by now and been widely adopted. However, we are where we are: further name changes are not warranted.

Instead, the global health community needs to work together to overcome the false dichotomies with the communicable and non-communicable labels and the perennial prevention versus treatment binary. Collectively we need to better market the construct we have, recognising its inherent inconsistencies, so as to increase understanding and awareness of the importance of the NCD agenda across governments and civil society so more appropriate funds are forthcoming and there is more pressure for action and tangible outcomes.

Rebooting the NCD agenda in the UN 2030 Agenda for Sustainable Development

Neither chronic NCDs nor mental health issues featured significantly in the Millenium Development Goals, resulting in them being rather invisible and often neglected elements of the global health agenda in the MDG era. Being underappreciated as development issues and underestimated as diseases with profound economic effects, governments in the global south had taken little interest in their prevention, leaving this responsibility primarily to individuals. With little attention given to chronic diseases, limited funding was devoted to their prevention and control. This indifference was unjustified and needed to be corrected (Beaglehole et al., 2007). It was imperative that NCDs figured prominently in the UN 2030 Agenda for Sustainable Development.

In 2014, the second HLM on NCDs comprehensively reviewed and assessed progress achieved in the prevention and control of NCDs. Ministers from around the world found progress was insufficient and highly uneven. While it saw no lack of commitment, it identified a lack of capacity to act across low- and middle-income countries from lack of access to expertise that was only generally available through international cooperation. The outcome document presented a focussed agenda for strengthening international cooperation: it agreed to give due consideration to addressing NCDs in the elaboration of the post-2015 development agenda, accepting that NCDs constitute one of the major challenges for development in the 21st century; and to take forward a proposed target to reduce premature mortality by one-third by 2030 (United Nations (UN), 2014).

This led in September 2015 to the inclusion of commitments, such as reducing premature mortality from NCDs and the promotion of physical activity, tobacco control, mental health and well-being in the UN 2030 Agenda for Sustainable Development: the agenda led to 17 separate but interlinked sustainable development goals (SDGs) which were adopted by 176 member states later that month. The aim is leaving no one behind and to reach the furthest behind first (United Nations (UN), 2015). The SDGs came with a complexity of 169 targets to be achieved by 2030, and 231 indicators to measure progress (Figure 6.1).

SDG Global Goal 3 is "good health and wellbeing". It has nine outcome targets and four means of achieving targets and 28 specific indicators to measure progress toward targets. Target 3.4 is to reduce by one-third premature mortality from NCDs through prevention and treatment by 2030 and to promote mental health and well-being. Several other targets are relevant to the NCD agenda: target 3.5 is to prevent and treat substance abuse, including the harmful use of alcohol; target 3.8 is to achieve UHC by 2030; target 3.9 is to reduce illnesses and deaths from hazardous chemicals and air pollution.

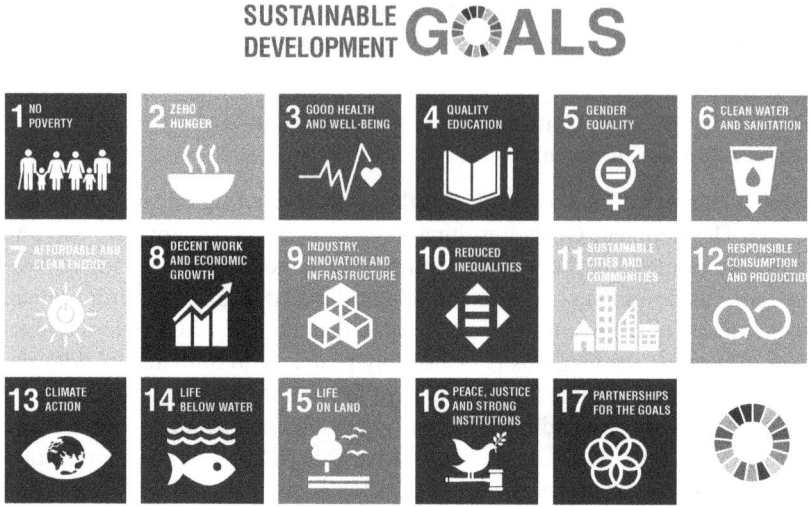

Figure 6.1 The 17 sustainable development goals

Three of four means of achieving the targets are of relevance to the NCD agenda: 3.a implement the WHO Framework Convention on Tobacco Control (FCTC); 3.b support research, development and universal access to affordable vaccines and medicines; and 3.c increase health financing and support health workforce in developing countries. These targets also interrelate to at least nine other SDG goals in addition to goal 3 (Thakur et al., 2021). All SDG targets are interlinked: targets 3.4 and 3.8 cannot be achieved if countries do not progress on both counts (Table 6.2).

Target 3.4 has two indicators: 3.4.1 is the mortality rate attributed to CVD, cancer, diabetes and chronic respiratory disease; 3.4.2 is the suicide mortality rate. Indicators for 3.5 are coverage of substance use disorders and harmful use of alcohol. Indicators for UHC are: 3.8.1, coverage of essential health services; and 3.8.2, proportion of population with large household expenditure on health. One indicator for pollution is 3.9.1, mortality from indoor, household and outdoor, ambient air pollution. For monitoring progress, baselines have to be established. The GBD 2017 study has attempted this and noted that it is increasingly important to go beyond national-level estimates to measure progress on health-related SDG indicators (Lozano et al., 2018).

In 2017, WHO established an independent high-level commission on NCDs that was charged with identifying innovative ways to curb the world's biggest causes of death and extend life expectancy for millions of people. It was designed to support political efforts to accelerate action on CVD, cancers, diabetes and respiratory diseases; to reduce suffering from mental health

Table 6.2 SDG 3 good health and well-being: nine targets and four means to achieve targets

Nine SDG 3 targets	Full text for the Individual targets to be achieved by 2030
Target 3.1: Reduce Maternal Mortality	By 2030, reduce the global maternity mortality ratio to less than 70 per 100,000 live births
Target 3.2: End all preventable deaths under five years of age	By 2030, end preventable deaths of newborns and children under 5 years of age with all countries aiming to reduce neonatal mortality below 12 per 1,000 live births and under-5 mortality under 25 per 1,000 live births
Target 3.3: Fight communicable diseases	By 2030, end the epidemics of AIDS, tuberculosis, malaria and neglected tropical diseases and combat hepatitis, water-borne diseases and other communicable diseases
Target 3.4: Reduce NCD mortality and promote mental health	By 2030, reduce by one-third premature mortality from non-communicable diseases through prevention and treatment and promote mental health and well-being
Target 3.5: Prevent and treat substance abuse	Strengthen the prevention and treatment of substance abuse, including narcotic drug abuse and harmful use of alcohol
Target 3.6: Reduce road injuries and deaths	By 2030, halve (50% less) the number of global deaths and injuries from road traffic accidents
Target 3.7: Universal access to sexual and reproductive care, and family planning	By 2030, ensure universal access to sexual and reproductive healthcare services, including for family planning, information and education and the integration of reproductive health into national strategies and programmes
Target 3.8: Achieve universal health coverage	Achieve universal health coverage, including financial risk protection, access to quality essential healthcare services and access to safe, effective, quality and affordable essential medicines and vaccines for all
Target 3.9: Reduce illness and death from pollution and hazardous chemicals	By 2030, substantially reduce the number of deaths and illnesses from hazardous chemicals and from air, water and soil pollution and from contamination

(Continued)

Table 6.2 (Continued)

Four means to achieve target	Full text for the means to achieve the nine targets
Target 3.a: Implement tobacco control	Strengthen the implementation of the WHO Framework Convention on Tobacco Control in all countries as appropriate
Target 3.b: Support research and development and universal access to vaccines and medicines	Support the research and development of vaccines and medicienes for the communicable and non-communicable diseases that primarily affect developing countries, provide access to affordable essential medicines and vaccines in accordance with the DOHA Declaration on the TRIPS Agreement and Public Health which affirms the right of developing countries to use the full provision in TRIPS regarding flexibilities to protect public health and in particular provide access to medicines for all
Target 3.c: Increase health financing and support health workforce development	Substantially increase health financing and the recruitment, development, training and retention of the health workforce in developing countries, especially the least developed countries and small island developing states
Target 3.d: Improve early warning systems for global health risks	Strengthen the capacity of all countries, in particular developing countries, for early warning, risk reduction and management of national and global health risks

conditions and to reduce the number of premature deaths from NCDs attributed to air pollution.

Its first report "Time to Deliver" identified several implementation issues including lack of political will and action, lack of policies and plans, difficulties in priority setting, lack of accountability and insufficient financing to scale up national NCD responses. The challenge is not only to gain political support but also to guarantee implementation, whether through legislation, norms and standard setting or investment (World Health Organization (WHO), 2018c).

A third UN HLM on the NCDs was held in October 2018, to accelerate progress to achieve SDG target 3.4 and to evolve the narrative from a disease-focussed perspective to a multistakeholder and cross-sectoral health and development perspective that better aligned with the SDG goals. The high-level commission on NCDs report was credited with the commitment made by Heads of State to scale up efforts against NCDs and mental health conditions by providing strategic leadership. This meeting also added mental health conditions and key environmental risk factors like air pollution to the NCD agenda (United Nations (UN), 2018).

Subsequently, the WHO Global Coordination Mechanism on the Prevention and Control of NCDs met in Geneva in late 2018. It highlighted the need to focus on greater country-level impact, grow its participant base and reach out to sectors other than health; and to find innovative ways to increase engagement with the private sector, particularly with industries beyond the pharmaceutical and nutrition sectors (World Health Organization (WHO), 2019a).

The final report of the High-level Commission on NCDs "Its Time to Walk the Talk" came out at the same time. It based its work on the common understanding reached at the UN General Assembly that the level of progress and investment to date was insufficient to meet SDG target 3.4; and that the world had still to fulfil its promise of implementing at all levels measures to reduce the risk of premature death and disability from NCDs. It underscored the need to greatly accelerate progress if the 2030 SDG agenda was to succeed and the essential promises to leave no-one behind and reach the furthest behind first was to be kept (World Health Organization (WHO), 2019b).

It has long been apparent that primary healthcare (PHC) will need to play a central role in the prevention and management of NCDs across the global south to achieve the 2030 target to reduce premature mortality by one-third. More people die from CVD worldwide than from any other cause. Policies and low-cost measures to reduce tobacco use, salt consumption and address other CVD risk factors are often underutilised in the global south meaning many people experience a CVD event.

In 2016 WHO and the US CDC launched the Global Hearts Initiative; on the management side it developed the HEARTS technical package aimed at strengthening the management of CVDs in PHC. Six HEARTS modules on healthy-lifestyle counselling, evidence-based protocols, access to essential CVD medicines and technology, risk-based CVD management, team-based care and systems for monitoring were produced. The target users at the PHC level were facility managers and trainers (World Health Organization (WHO), 2018b).

In 2020, WHO widened its guidance around a prioritised set of cost-effective essential interventions for primary care that were able to deliver an acceptable quality of care in low-resource settings. The package for essential non-communicable (PEN) disease interventions defined a minimum set of interventions to address major NCDs in primary care. The interventions are for the detection, diagnosis, treatment and care of CVD, diabetes and chronic respiratory diseases; early cancer diagnosis; and core components of healthy lifestyle, self-care and palliative care.

All are considered feasible and able to be delivered by primary care physicians and non-physician health workers. The clinical pathways all include referral to a higher level of care for further management of complications. Countries can expand on the core interventions according to their needs and resources: content can be adapted to emergency and humanitarian settings (World Health Organization (WHO), 2020).

In 2021, WHO updated information about NCDs in a summary fact sheet: NCDs kill over 40 million people each year, equivalent to at least 70% of all deaths globally. They disproportionately affect people in low- and middle-income countries where more than three quarters of global NCD deaths occur: most are considered premature occurring between the ages of 30 and 69. Four groups of diseases account for almost all premature NCD deaths: CVDs (such as heart attacks and stroke); cancers; chronic respiratory diseases, such as asthma and chronic obstructive pulmonary disease and diabetes (World Health Organization (WHO), 2022a).

The NCDs share key modifiable behavioural risk factors like tobacco use, unhealthy diet, lack of physical activity, excess salt intake and the harmful use of alcohol which in turn lead to overweight and obesity, raised blood pressure, raised cholesterol and ultimately disease and premature death. Two priority cancers, cervical and liver, are vaccine-preventable. Effective interventions like obesity management and smoking cessation and effective therapies to control raised blood glucose, elevated blood pressure and hyperlipidaemia are widely available and used in the global north to prevent disease, reduce morbidity and premature mortality.

Most recently, WHO has published a report to advance the global NCD agenda on the prevention and control of NCDs which looks forward to 2030. The document recalled political commitments made by heads of state and governments at the UN; and outlined and updated the technical guidance provided by WHO towards achieving the 2030 SDG target. It highlighted the landmarks and key milestones in the development and implementation of the global agenda for NCDs over the last two decades. It summarised where the world was in 2000, where it is in 2022, and where it wants to be in terms of NCD prevention and control by 2030. The 2013 GAP was extended to 2030 and its nine voluntary global NCD targets were updated (Table 6.3).

WHO reiterated that at a global level, seven of the ten leading causes of death in 2019 were NCDs; and that premature deaths, occurring between the ages of 30 and 70 when people are most economically productive were rapidly increasing. It reinforced the need to track the implementation of the GAP across its six objectives, ten progress monitoring indicators. It committed WHO to report on progress towards SDG target 3.4, the reduction of premature NCD mortality by one-third, to the WHA and the UN in 2025 and 2030 (World Health Organization (WHO), 2023a).

Table 6.3 The nine updated voluntary global targets for the NCDs

NCD framework element	Updated (2023) voluntary NCD target
Premature morbidity and mortality from NCDs	A one-third reduction in the probability of dying between the ages of 30 and 70 from CVDs, cancer, diabetes or chronic respiratory diseases by 2030 *(changed from a 25% relative reduction in overall mortality)*
Behavioural risk factors	A 20% relative reduction in the harmful use of alcohol by 2030 *(changed from at least a 10% relative reduction)*
Behavioural risk factors	A 15% relative reduction in prevalence of insufficient physical activity by 2030 *(changed from a 10% relative reduction)*
Behavioural risk factors	A 30% relative reduction in mean population intake of salt/sodium by 2030 *(unchanged from 2025 target)*
Behavioural risk factors	A 30% relative reduction in the prevalence of current tobacco use by 2030 *(unchanged from 2025 target)*
Premature morbidity and mortality from NCDs	A 25% relative reduction in prevalence of raised blood pressure or to contain prevalence of raised blood pressure by 2030 *(unchanged from 2025 target)*
Premature morbidity and mortality from NCDs	Halt the rise in diabetes and obesity by 2030 *(unchanged from 2025 target)*
Premature morbidity and mortality from NCDs	At least 50% of eligible people (40 years and older with a 10-year cardiovascular risk over 20%) including those with CVD to receive drug therapy and counselling (including glycaemic control) to prevent heart attacks and strokes *(unchanged from 2025 target)*
Premature morbidity and mortality from NCDs	An 80% availability of the affordable basic technologies and essential medicines including generics, required to treat major NCDs in both public and private facilities by 2030 *(unchanged from 2025 target)*

The nine global NCD targets for 2025 in 2013 WHO NCD Global Action Plan were updated in 2023 Advancing the global agenda on prevention and control of NCDs: looking forward to 2030.

The report also highlighted the two global health movements that have helped shape the pathways to prevention and control of NCDs and helped to steer the associated political agenda. One is the focus on PHC and the other is the pursuit of UHC.

• PHC is the most effective, efficient and equitable way to improve health across the life course. Comprehensive NCD management requires assessment of risk factors, early detection of high-risk status or disease, a combination of behavioural and pharmacological treatment, long-term follow-up with regular monitoring and promotion of adherence that requires a comprehensive PHC approach.

- UHC ensures that all people have access to needed health services including prevention, promotion, treatment, rehabilitation and palliation; and are of sufficient quality to be effective whilst also ensuring that the use of these services does not expose the user to financial hardship.

Delivering on SDG target 3.8, to achieve UHC by 2030, reinforces the delivery of the NCD agenda by ensuring universal access to nationally determined sets of integrated, quality health services at all levels of care for prevention, diagnosis, treatment and care in a timely manner.

7 Unpacking the chronic non-communicable diseases agenda

The main groups of diseases in the NCD construct

Contrary to how it may seem, there is no one single fixed list of what diseases constitute the chronic non-communicable diseases (NCDs); nor how many major different NCD groupings there are. Five groups are generally used: cardiovascular diseases (CVDs); chronic respiratory diseases (CRDs); cancers; diabetes and mental health and disorders. They share five risk factors making what is now called the five-by-five approach NCD control This has not always been the case (Figure 7.1).

The WHO Global Action Plan (GAP) for the Prevention and Control of NCDs 2013–2020 had four disease groups and four risk factors, with nine global NCD targets to be attained by 2025, including a 25% relative reduction in premature mortality from NCDs by 2025, often referred to as "25 by 25" (World Health Organization (WHO), 2013). The third UN HLM on NCDs in September 2018 signalled a shift from the four-by-four approach to a five-by-five response, adding a fifth disease group, mental health and neurological conditions, and a fifth shared risk factor, key environmental risk factors particularly air pollution, to the list (United Nations (UN), 2018).

WHO subsequently updated the NCD GAP to include air pollution; extended the plan to 2030; and aligned its target with SDG target 3.4 "to reduce by one-third premature mortality from NCDs through prevention and treatment by 2030" (World Health Organization (WHO), 2023a). But WHO has not formally added mental health to the four NCD disease groups outlined in its GAP (Banatvala et al., 2023).

Cardiovascular diseases: the five globally most important CVDs by incidence and disease burden are in rank order: ischaemic heart disease, disease of the blood vessels that supply the heart; cerebrovascular disease, which is divided by GBD into haemorrhagic/other strokes and ischaemic stroke; hypertensive heart disease largely heart failure and arterial disease as the heart works harder raising blood pressure; cardiomyopathy and myocarditis, diseases of the heart muscle; and rheumatic heart disease, a sequela of childhood streptococcal pharyngitis. In

DOI: 10.4324/9781003505693-10

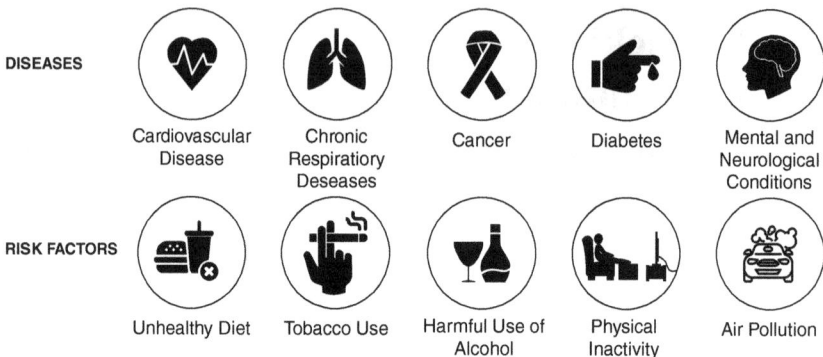

Figure 7.1 The five-by-five approach to the NCDs

percentage terms these five diseases make up 95% of all CVD deaths. Smoking, alcohol, hypertension, diabetes and obesity are some of the important modifiable risk factors (Joseph et al., 2017).

Chronic respiratory diseases: the four leading CRDs globally are chronic obstructive pulmonary disease (COPD), asthma and rhinitis, occupational lung disease and sleep-disordered breathing. A billion people globally are estimated to suffer from them, the majority living in the global south. The CRDs have major adverse effects on life and disability; and together they are the third leading cause of NCD deaths. The main risk factors for CRDs include tobacco smoking, indoor air pollution and particularly biomass fuel combustion, outdoor air pollution, unhealthy diet and obesity, allergen and toxic occupational exposures (Bousquet et al., 2010).

Diabetes: diabetes affects half a billion people globally, 80% of whom live in low- and middle-income countries. There are two types of diabetes; elevated blood sugar, the hallmark of diabetes, can also occur during pregnancy when it is called gestational diabetes. Type 1 diabetes commonly occurs in childhood or adolescence. Insulin production is impaired and daily insulin injections are needed to control blood sugar levels and avoid late-stage complications. Type 2 diabetes is more common in adults and accounts for over 90% of diabetes cases globally. Insulin is produced but it is not well used by the cells in the body and blood sugar levels are persistently elevated. The cornerstone of type 2 diabetes prevention and management is a healthy lifestyle including increased physical activity and a healthy diet. Over time most people with type 2 diabetes will require treatment with oral medicines or insulin for glycaemic control (Roglic, 2016).

Cancer: cancer is a heterogeneous disease with numerous different types and forms that vary significantly in their incidence and prevalence, aetiology, pathology and geographical distribution. Geographical variations in cancer arise because risk factor exposure differs in given populations. Priorities for cancer prevention, screening and diagnosis and treatment need to be developed at regional and national levels to accommodate this heterogeneity. Although the rank orders differ by region, six cancers predominate: breast, lung, cervix, liver, colorectum and prostate. Smoking is a major risk factor for most cancers along with alcohol, poor diet, physical inactivity, obesity and chronic viral infection, with hepatitis B or C viruses and human papilloma virus (HPV) (Wild, 2012).

Mental health: mental health is a global public good and is relevant to sustainable development in all countries. The main mental health disorders include substance use, addiction to drugs and alcohol, self-harm and dementia. The global burden of mental health disorders has risen in all countries but the quality of mental health services is routinely worse than the quality of those for physical health (Patel et al., 2018). WHO emphasised a separate focus on mental health and disorders in its updated comprehensive mental health action plan 2013–2030. Good mental health is essential for all to lead fulfilling lives, to participate productively in society and to demonstrate resilience in the face of stress and adversity; mental health services are an essential component of healthcare and UHC. Health systems have not adequately responded to the burden of mental disorders: between 76% and 85% of people in low- and middle-income countries with severe disorders receive no treatment. Countries are urged to integrate mental health into primary healthcare (PHC). Mental health and neurological conditions are seen by WHO as a core component of the PHC and UHC agendas rather than a specific part of the NCD response (World Health Organization (WHO), 2021a).

Seven of the ten leading causes of death in 2019 were NCDs: 15 of 36 million deaths were regarded as premature; 85% of the premature deaths from NCDs occurred in low- and middle-income countries. Most premature deaths are preventable (World Health Organization (WHO), 2023a):

- Two cardiovascular diseases, ischaemic heart disease and strokes, are the top leading global causes of premature mortality, deaths in those aged between 30 and 70 years: in 2019, over 6 million CVD deaths occurred, 40% of global premature deaths.
- In the same period, cancers at 31% were the second leading cause of death with just under five million premature deaths: lung cancer was the most prevalent.
- CRDs were the third leading cause at 7% with just over a million deaths: chronic obstructive pulmonary disease was the leading CRD.
- Diabetes, particularly type 2, was the fourth leading cause at 4% causing just under one million premature deaths.
- Mental health and neurological conditions were the fifth leading cause at around 3% and responsible for around 600,000 premature deaths.
- In 2019, kidney disease was the tenth leading global cause of death.

All groups working on NCD prevention and control have aligned around SDG target 3.4 to reduce by one-third premature mortality from NCDs through prevention and treatment by 2030; but often have not included the second part, the promotion of mental health and are not routinely tracking its indicator, the suicide mortality rate.

While many have adopted the five-by-five approach, some groups have continued to see a cluster of four NCD groups: for example, NCD countdown 2030 considers cancers, CVD, CRD and diabetes without mental health and disorders noting that in 2016 deaths from these four disease groups comprised 80% of NCD deaths, estimated to be 32.2 million (Bennett et al., 2018).

The WHO PEN package of essential NCD interventions for PHC focusses on CVD, diabetes, CRD and cancer early diagnosis and notes that mental health is covered in the mental health action plan; it also has components of healthy lifestyle counselling, self-care and palliative care in the package (World Health Organization (WHO), 2020).

Others have a broader view of NCDs and the linkage with UHC. The third edition of the World Bank Disease Control Priorities (DCP3) enterprise was built around 21 essential packages grouped into four clusters with a mix of intersectoral policies and health-sector interventions: an age-related cluster; an infectious diseases cluster; an NCD and injury cluster; and a health services cluster. The NCD and injury cluster has seven packages: cardiovascular, respiratory and related disorders; cancer; mental, neurological and substance use disorders; musculoskeletal disorders; congenital and generic disorders; injury prevention; and environmental improvements. It defined a model concept of essential universal health coverage (EUHC) which had 218 interventions that provide a starting point for country-specific analysis of disease priorities (Jamison et al., 2018).

There are other NCD groups and conditions which could be included. Chronic kidney disease (CKD) is widely prevalent, harmful and treatable and is a leading cause of premature death. It is both a major contributing factor to the incidence and outcome of diabetes and cardiovascular diseases; and a major risk factor for CVD, particularly through raised blood pressure. The GBD 2019 study noted that CKD is in the top 20 of leading causes of disability-adjusted life years (DALYs). Kidney disease in 2019 was the tenth leading cause of death. However, kidney disease does not figure in the current taxonomy of NCDs as a separate major disease group. In WHO PEN, it is subsumed into the diabetes and CVD risk assessment and management sections; its diagnosis and management is not considered a best buy or a recommended intervention for the prevention and control of NCDs.

Obesity may need to be considered for inclusion as a major disease group. It is widely seen as a disease in its own right, with both genetic and environmental determinants; and is now the fastest-growing epidemic in many high- and low-income countries. It has been grouped together with undernutrition and climate change as a global syndemic, which represents the paramount health challenge for humans, the environment and our planet in the 21st century (Swinburn et al., 2019). It is a major contribution to premature mortality by itself with its own ICD codes, as well as being a significant risk factor for three major NCD groups – diabetes, cardiovascular disease and cancer. There are both surgical and therapeutic interventions for the treatment of obesity (Bray, 2006).

Both GBD and DCP recognise that there are several conditions including mental disorders, genetic diseases, disabilities, violence and injuries that figure in the wider NCD construct; that contribute significantly to global morbidity and are disease control priorities for many countries; but that have a lesser impact on global premature mortality that the four initial major NCD groupings.

One single action plan that addresses all the important NCDs and the priority causes of premature morbidity in equal detail would be unwieldly and difficult to implement. For this reason, WHO sticks to a simpler approach with four major NCD groups with shared actions for prevention and control in the GAP for the prevention and control of NCDs.

The five shared NCD risk factors and interventions that address them

In contrast to the complexity of the NCD construct and the various ways they have been grouped together for concerted and coherent action planning, the different major risk factors are easier to describe and group together into five major thematic areas that nicely fit into the five-by-five agenda: tobacco use; unhealthy diet; harmful use of alcohol; physical activity; and air pollution.

There are several different interventions and overarching policy actions for NCD prevention and control in each of these key risk factor grouping that all link together. While some NCD risk factors imply personal behaviours and impact at the individual level, national public policies in sectors like trade, taxation, pharmaceuticals, tobacco, food production, urban development, health education and health promotion have a major bearing on reducing risks for NCDs at the population level; and are often synergistic and cross-cutting, impacting several NCD groups.

For many years, WHO has promoted a stepwise approach to surveillance (STEPS) of risk factors for chronic NCDs to support countries in the global south to develop primary prevention interventions. There was concern that if the rapid increase in NCDs was left uncontrolled there would be significant social, economic and health consequences which in turn would overwhelm already overstretched health services. It noted that the emerging major risk factors for the most common and important NCDs – tobacco and alcohol use, physical inactivity, high blood pressure and high cholesterol – are all amenable to prevention.

The key information required for planning primary preventative programmes and for helping predict the future caseload of NCDs is the population distribution of the major common risk factors (Bonita et al., 2003). A manual was produced to provide guidelines and supporting material for sites embarking on STEPS chronic disease risk factor surveillance: this helped countries plan and prepare the survey, train staff, conduct the survey, capture and analyse the data collected and report and disseminate the results (World Health Organization (WHO), 2005b).

In 2017, WHO produced an influential document that provided national policymakers with a list of "best buys" and other recommended interventions for the prevention and control of NCDs and to help reduce premature NCD deaths in the global south. It listed 88 interventions that ranged across overarching enabling policy actions, cost-effective interventions and other recommended actions: the 16 best buys were identified through a combination of cost-effectiveness analysis, likely health impact and costs of implementation. The best buys have an average cost-effectiveness of $100 or less per disability-adjusted life-year (DALY) averted in low- and middle-income countries. It may need to be updated with more data and to include mental health and air pollution (Table 7.1).

The economic analyses that identify cost-effective interventions have all been performed using data from studies conducted in situations where there are reasonably well-functioning health systems or policy environments for effective implementation: if systems are performing below this level then the interventions may be compromised and their efficiency may well not be realised. This important caveat about the assumptions and limitations of cost-effectiveness analysis (CEA) was emphasised by the DCP project, one of the pioneers of CEA in the global south to help prioritise which disease control activities to concentrate on (Laxminarayan et al., 2006).

Many countries have used the list of best buys and other recommended interventions to develop national plans and policies for NCD control. When considering the interventions that will bring the highest return on investment countries need to give attention to non-economic criteria along with the CEA data as both will affect implementation and impact. Important issues, such as equity, community acceptability, health impact, scalability and sustainability together with practical considerations, such as feasibility, work-force skills and capacity and, the suitability of existing rural and urban facilities are all important to consider (World Health Organization (WHO), 2017).

The majority of best buy and other interventions aim at reducing modifiable risk factors for NCD and underlying social determinants through intersectoral health-promoting policy and the creation of healthy environments. They are listed around the five major risk factors:

Tobacco use is generally regarded as the most pernicious and important risk factor for the NCDs; and is one of the biggest global public health threats, being responsible for untold morbidity and over 8 million preventable deaths a year. In February 2005, the WHO Framework Convention on Tobacco Control (FTCT), an evidence-based legally binding instrument with a core set of mutually reinforcing

Table 7.1 The 16 "best buy" policy or clinical interventions for NCD control

NCD objective	Best buy intervention
Tobacco control	# Increased excise taxes and prices on tobacco products # Plain packaging and large graphic health warnings on all packages # Enact and enforce comprehensive bans on tobacco advertising, promotion and sponsorship # Eliminate exposure to second-hand tobacco smoke in all indoor workplaces, public places, public transport # Implement effective mass media campaigns that educate the public about the harms of smoking and second-hand smoke
Harmful use of alcohol	# Increase excise taxes on alcoholic beverages # Enact and enforce bans or restrictions on exposure to alcohol advertising across multiple types of media # Enact and enforce restrictions on the physical availability of retailed alcohol (via reduces hours of sale)
Unhealthy diets	# Reduce salt intake through the reformulation of food products to contain less salt and set target levels for the amount of salt in food # Reduce salt intake through supportive environments in public institutions such as hospitals, schools, workplaces and nursing homes # Reduce salt intake through behaviour change communication and mass media campaigns # Reduce salt intake through implementation of front-of-pack labels
Physical inactivity	# Implement community-wide public education and awareness campaign for physical activity which includes a mass media campaign combined with other community-based education, motivational and environmental programmes aimed at supporting behaviour change of physical activity levels
Manage cardiovascular disease and diabetes	# Drug therapy (including glycaemic control for diabetes mellitus and control of hypertension using a total risk approach) and counselling to individuals who have had a heart attack or stroke and to persons with a high risk (>30%) of a fatal and non-fatal cardiovascular event in the next ten years
Manage cancer	# Vaccinate against human papillomavirus (with 2 doses) of 9–13 year old girls # Prevention of cervical cancer by screening women aged 30–49 linked with timely treatment of pre-cancerous lesions either through visual inspection, Pap smear or HPV test every 5 years

These are considered the most cost-effective and feasible for implementation in low and lower middle-income countries.

obligations to reduce the demand for and supply of tobacco products came into force: by June 2023, 182 ember states had become parties to the Convention.

A technical package was designed to catalyse global action on tobacco control: MPOWER identifies six broad measures for effective tobacco control: *mon*itor tobacco use and prevention policies; *p*rotect people from tobacco smoke; *o*ffer help to quit tobacco use; *w*arn about dangers of tobacco; *e*nforce bans on tobacco advertising, promotion and sponsorship; and *r*aise taxes on tobacco. All measures are evidence-based and cost-effective across all country income levels. WHO regularly produces a report on the global tobacco epidemic which includes progress that has been achieved and challenges that remain in MPOWER implementation (World Health Organization (WHO), 2023e).

Five MPOWER measures are recognised by WHO as NCD best buy interventions, with CEA less than $100 per DALY averted in low- and middle-income countries:

1 Increase excise taxes and prices on tobacco products
2 Plain/standardised packaging and/or large graphic health warnings on all tobacco packages
3 Enact and enforce comprehensive bans on tobacco advertising, promotion and sponsorship
4 Eliminate exposure to second-hand tobacco smoke in all indoor workplaces, public places and public transport
5 Implement effective mass media campaigns that educate the public about the harms of smoking/tobacco use and second-hand smoke.

A sixth intervention is regarded as cost-effective, with a CEA over $100 per DALY averted: to provide cost-covered, effective, population-wide support (including advice and toll-free quit line services) for tobacco cessation to all who want to quit. Three further activities are recommended but do not have CEA data to rank them: implement measures to minimise illicit trade in tobacco products; ban cross-border advertising, including modern means of communication; provide mobile phone-based cessation services for all those who want to quit.

Reducing unhealthy diets links with the overarching action to implement the global strategy on diet, physical activity and health; and WHO recommendations on marketing of foods and non-alcoholic beverages to children. Several top interventions relate to salt intake because of the long-recognised association of high dietary salt intake and population prevalence of hypertension in most societies (Karppanen & Mervaala, 2006). Dietary fatty acids play significant roles in the cause and prevention of CVD: trans fatty acids from partially hydrogenated vegetable oils have well-established adverse effects and should be eliminated from the human diet; the moderate CVD risks from saturated fatty acids can be ameliorated by unsaturated dietary fatty acids (Michas et al., 2014).

There is a clear, strong benefit from taxing sugar-sweetened beverages to help reduce excess sugar consumption (Brownell et al., 2009). Exclusive breastfeeding is important especially for the first six months of life. Healthy diets should be promoted, including higher intake of fruit and vegetables with smaller portion sizes to reduce obesity. Food labelling has an increasingly recognised role in supporting consumer choice and healthy diets.

Four healthy diet interventions are recognised as NCD best buys:

1 Reduce salt intake through the reformulation of food products to contain less salt and the setting of target levels for the amount of salt in food and meals.
2 Reduce salt intake by establishing a supportive environment in public institutions, such as hospitals, schools, workplaces and nursing homes to provide lower sodium options.
3 Reduce salt intake through a behaviour change communication and mass media campaign.
4 Reduce salt intake through the implementation of front-of-pack labelling.

Two further dietary interventions are regarded as cost-effective, with a CEA over $100 per DALY averted: the elimination of industrial trans-fats through the development of legislation to ban their use in the food chain; and the reduction of sugar consumption through effective taxation on sugar-sweetened beverages. Several other interventions are recommended but do not have CEA data to rank them: the promotion of breastfeeding for the first six months of life; the replacement of trans-fats and saturated fats with unsaturated fats; the use of subsidies to increase the intake of fruits and vegetables; limiting portion size to reduce energy intake and the risk of overweight/obesity; better nutrition labelling to reduce total energy intake, sugars, sodium and fats; mass media campaigns on health diets, social marketing to reduce the intake of total fats, sugar and salt and to promote fruits and vegetables; the implementation of nutrition education and counselling especially in schools.

The harmful use of alcohol seriously impacts public health and is a major risk factor for poor health and mental disorders globally. The concept of harmful alcohol use is broad and encompasses the drinking that causes detrimental health and social consequences for the drinker, the people around the drinker and socially at large. It is a major avoidable risk factor for neuropsychiatric disorders, cardiovascular disease, chronic liver damage and cirrhosis and several cancers, including liver and stomach. Harms include unintentional and intentional injuries, road traffic accidents, violence and suicide; fatal injuries tend to occur in relatively young people.

A substantial evidence base exists for policymakers on the costs and effectiveness of strategies and interventions to prevent and reduce alcohol-related harm. Data largely come from high-income settings: meta-analysis and reviews of evidence provide sufficient knowledge to inform policy recommendations in the global south and at regional as well as national level (World Health Organization (WHO), 2010).

Three interventions to combat the harmful use of alcohol are recognised as NCD best buys:

1 The increase of excise taxes on alcoholic beverages.
2 Enact and enforce bans or comprehensive restrictions on exposure to alcohol advertising across multiple types of media.
3 Enact and enforce restrictions on the physical availability of retailed alcohol via reduced hours of sale.

Two further interventions are recognised as cost-effective with a CEA over $100 per DALY averted: the enactment and enforcement of drink-driving laws and blood alcohol concentrations limits via sobriety checkpoints; the provision of brief psychosocial interventions for persons with hazardous and harmful alcohol use. Several other interventions are recommended but do not have CEA data to rank them: regular review of prices in relation to inflation and income; establish a minimum price for alcohol; enact and enforce an appropriate minimum age for alcohol purchase and consumption; ban or restrict the promotion of alcoholic beverages targeting young people; provide treatment and care for alcohol use disorders and comorbid conditions in health and social services; provide consumer information and label alcoholic beverages to indicate the harm related to alcohol.

Physical activity has an important role in the promotion of health mental well-being and maintaining a healthy lifestyle. Much epidemiological evidence, primarily from high-income settings, supports a strong independent and inverse association between physical activity and the fitness status of an individual and mortality in apparently healthy individuals and diseased populations; and is supported by evidence from intervention studies. The health benefits start at low fitness levels and increase with higher physical activity patterns or fitness status in a dose-dependent fashion. Risk reduction is partly attributed to the favourable effect of exercise and physical activity on CVD risk factors, blood pressure, diabetes and obesity (Kokkinos et al., 2011).

One intervention increased physical activity is recognised as an NCD best buy:

1 Implement community-wide public education and awareness campaign for physical activity which includes a mass media campaign with community-based education, motivational and environmental programmes to support behavioural change of physical activity levels.

One further intervention is recognised as cost-effective with a CEA over $100 per DALY averted: the provision of physical activity counselling and referral as part of routine PHC services through the use of a brief intervention. Several other interventions are recommended but do not have CEA data to rank them: ensure that macro-level urban design incorporates the core elements of residential density, connected street networks, easy access to a diversity of destinations and access to public transport; implement whole-of-school programmes that include quality physical education, availability of adequate facilities and programmes to support physical activities for all children; provide convenient safe access to quality public open space and adequate infrastructure to support walking and cycling; implement multi-component workplace physical activity programmes; promotion of physical activity through organised sport groups and clubs.

Air pollution was added as the fifth, and main environmental risk factor following the third UN HLM on NCDS in 2018 and thus does not figure in the WHO best buys list for tackling NCDs, published in 2017. Adding this opened up the focus of risk factors from the behavioural to a wider consideration of environmental determinants of health including indoor and outdoor air pollution, water and soil pollution and climate change. The epidemiological imperative to address air pollution is irrefutable: it is associated with over five million NCD deaths annually and is strongly linked to CVD, CRD and lung cancer deaths (Linou et al., 2018).

Clinical management interventions for NCD prevention and control

A much smaller number of best buy and other interventions aim to strengthen and orient health systems to address the prevention and control of NCDs and the underlying social determinants through people-centred PHC and universal health coverage. They are listed below around clinical services for managing CVD and diabetes; managing diabetes; managing cancer; and mental health.

Managing CVD and diabetes: Screening for diabetes by measuring blood sugar, or for cardiovascular disease risk factors like high blood pressure or high cholesterol identifies individuals who will benefit from drug treatment to reduce the risk factor identified so as to prevent diabetic complications or cardiovascular events like stroke from developing. Screening to identify asymptomatic individuals without prior disease for treatment to stop disease from appearing is primary prevention; treating individuals after a heart attack or stroke to stop recurrent disease is secondary prevention. Using therapeutic interventions can be seen as biomedical prevention as opposed to biobehavioural prevention like eating healthily, regularly exercising, reducing alcohol use or stopping smoking.

One intervention to manage cardiovascular disease and diabetes is recognised as an NCD best buy:

1 Drug therapy (including glycaemic control for diabetes and control of hypertension using a total risk approach) and counselling to individuals who have had a heart attack or stroke and to persons with >30% risk of a fatal or non-fatal cardiovascular event in the next ten years.

Several clinical management interventions are recognised as cost-effective with a CEA over $100 per DALY averted: treatment of new cases of acute myocardial infarction (MI) in hospital with aspirin alone or with clopidogrel to stop platelets sticking together and forming clots; thrombolysis or primary percutaneous coronary intervention with follow up carried out through PHC facilities at a 95% coverage rate; treatment of ischaemic stroke with intravenous thrombolytic therapy in hospitals with capacity to diagnose ischaemic stroke; primary prevention of rheumatic fever and rheumatic heart disease by increasing appropriate treatment of streptococcal pharyngitis at the primary care level; and secondary prevention of rheumatic fever and rheumatic heart disease by developing a register of patients for regular prophylactic penicillin. Several other interventions are recommended but do not have CEA data to rank them: treating congestive cardiac failure with angiotensin-converting-enzyme (ACE) inhibitor, beta-blocker and diuretic; cardiac rehabilitation post-MI; anticoagulation for medium- and high-risk non-valvular atrial fibrillation and for mitral stenosis with atrial fibrillation; low-dose aspirin for ischaemic stroke; care and rehabilitation in stroke units.

Managing diabetes: No highly cost-effective NCD best buy interventions are identified for diabetes management alone; there is one included above with CVD management when glycaemic control is provided with treatment to reduce blood pressure.

Several clinical management interventions are recognised as cost-effective with a CEA over $100 per DALY averted: preventive foot care for diabetic patients, which needs record systems for patient recall; diabetic retinopathy screening for all diabetes patients and laser photocoagulation for the prevention of blindness which also needs systems for patient follow-up and recall; effective glycaemic control for people with diabetes along with standard home glucose monitoring for people treated with insulin to reduce complications. Several other interventions are recommended but do not have CEA data to rank them: lifestyle interventions for preventing type 2 diabetes; influenza vaccination for diabetic patients; preconception care among women of reproductive age who have diabetes, including patient education and intensive blood sugar management; screening of diabetic patients for proteinuria and treatment with ACE inhibitors for the prevention and delay of CKD.

Managing cancer: some common cancers are caused by viruses and are vaccine-preventable. Cancer management interventions relate to the types of cancer that are prevalent in a country or region, and in many cases require access to second-level hospitals which can offer surgery, radiotherapy and chemotherapy services. When cancer surveillance is limited and patients present with very late disease, or specialist hospital clinical management is not readily accessible, patients will still benefit from palliative and end-of-life care.

Two clinical interventions to prevent cancer are recognised as NCD best buys:

1 Vaccination against HPV of 9–13 year old girls with two doses.
2 Prevention of cervical cancer by screening women aged 30–49 through visual inspection of the cervix, pap smear every 3–5 years or HPV test every five years all then linked with timely referral for treatment of precancerous lesions.

Several clinical interventions for the management of cancer are recognised as cost-effective with a CEA over $100 per DALY averted: mammography once every two years for women aged 50–69, with timely diagnosis and treatment of breast cancer; treatment of colorectal cancer with surgery and/or chemotherapy and radiotherapy; treatment of early stages of cervical cancer with surgery and/ or chemotherapy; treatment of early-stage breast cancer with surgery and/or systemic therapy; basic palliative care for cancer, home-based and hospital care with multidisciplinary teams and access to opiate and essential supportive medicines for pain relief. Several interventions are recommended but do not have CEA data to rank them: prevention of liver cancer through hepatitis B immunisation; oral cancer screening in high-risk groups like tobacco users and betel nut chewers, linked with timely treatment; and population-based colorectal cancer screening including through a faecal occult blood test at age over 50 with timely treatment.

One tobacco control intervention that is important in lung cancer prevention can also be considered a clinical management intervention: provide cost-covered, effective, population-wide support for tobacco cessation to all who want to quit smoking. One of the mainstays in smoking cessation is nicotine replacement therapy (NRT) which aims to replace the addictive nicotine in carcinogenic tobacco smoke with substitute nicotine in skin patches, inhalers or vaporised in electronic devises.

Managing mental health and disorders: Mental health is the unique interplay of environmental and social influences interacting with genetic, neurodevelopmental and psychological processes. Mental health conditions exist on a continuum from mild, time-limited distress to chronic, progressive and severely disabling: a binary diagnostic approach useful for clinical practice does not readily reflect the diversity or complexity of population mental health needs. Common problems include substance use disorders (alcohol and drugs), self-harm and dementia, increasing globally as populations age.

Mental health is a fundamental human right that requires a rights-based approach to protect the welfare of people with mental disorders and those with poor mental health and to ensure they have access to appropriate services for mental healthcare. The global burden of mental health disorders has risen in all countries but the quality of mental health services is routinely worse than the quality of those for physical health. SDG 3 indicators for mental health include 3.4.2, suicide mortality rate; 3.5.1, coverage of treatment interventions for substance use disorders; 3.5.2, harmful use of alcohol; 3.8.1, coverage of essential health services (Patel et al., 2018).

The WHO Comprehensive Mental Health Action Plan 2013–2030 has a series of actions to promote mental health and well-being for all, to prevent mental health conditions from developing in those at risk and to achieve universal coverage for mental health services. It noted that health systems have not yet adequately responded to the burden of mental disorders: between 76% and 85% of people in low- and middle-income countries with severe disorders receive no treatment for their disorder.

Three targets to improve mental health and social care services access by 2030 were proposed: service coverage for mental health conditions to increase at least by 50%; 80% of countries will have doubled the number of community-based mental health facilities; and 80% of countries will have integrated mental health into primary care. No specific cost-effectiveness analysis of intersectoral policies or health-sector interventions have been conducted to help guide countries towards which actions to address mental disorders may be best buys or give the highest return on investment (World Health Organization (WHO), 2021a).

Implementing NCD control interventions: government leadership and political will

Many commentators have emphasised the importance of the political process in addressing the NCD epidemic and committing to effective NCD prevention and control measures, with some suggesting that the collective failure to address the chronic disease pandemic in the early 2000s was a political rather than a technical failure (Geneau et al., 2010). Much of the work leading up to the UN HLMs on NCDs focussed on member states making political commitments to act on the NCDs; and then to the SDGs and the commitment to reducing premature NCD mortality (United Nations (UN), 2015).

The WHO Independent High-level Commission on NCDs recognised that the challenge is not only to gain political support but also to guarantee implementation, whether through legislation, norms and standards setting or investment. It integrated and synthesised government commitments made in 2011 and 2014 at UN HLMs into a new set of recommendations for member states to drive the NCD agenda forward (World Health Organization (WHO), 2018c). These remain clear and relevant today.

Heads of state and government, not Ministers of health only, should oversee the process of creating ownership at the national level of NCDs and mental health. Political leaders at all levels should take responsibility for comprehensive local actions, together with the health sector, that can advance action. Governments should identify and implement a specific set of priorities within the overall NCD and mental health agenda based on public health needs.

A series of strong recommendations were made about packages and services; and their integrated delivery. Governments should ensure that the national UHC public benefit package includes NCD and mental health services, including health promotion and prevention and priority healthcare interventions as well as access to essential medicines and technologies. PHC services should be strengthened to ensure equitable coverage including essential public health functions with an adequate and multidisciplinary health workforce. Synergies should be identified in existing chronic-care platforms, such as HIV and TB to help jumpstart NCD and mental health services.

Areas where governments should take the lead in planning and policy-making were identified:

- the creation of health-protecting environments through robust laws and through dialogue based on the "health is the priority" principle
- constructive engagement with the private sector, except tobacco, to strengthen action and commitments to achieving public health goals in accordance with the SDG mandate
- manage commercial and other vested interests from the food, alcohol and soft drinks companies in policy areas, such as reformulating, labelling and regulating markets
- restrict the marketing of unhealthy products (those with excess sodium, sugar, saturated and trans-fats) particularly to children, ideally through partnerships based on aligned interests rather than policy edicts
- work with the leisure and sports industries to promote physical activity; and the transport sector to ensure safe, clean and sustainable mobility
- providing incentives to encourage healthy lifestyles
- work with the pharmaceutical industry and vaccine manufacturers to ensure access to affordable, quality-assured essential medicines and vaccines
- ensure the meaningful engagement and participation of civil society and PLWNCDs and seek to strengthen alliances with civil society and NCD pressure groups
- work with civil society and people with mental conditions to effectively end discrimination and human rights violations and to plan and implement mental health services.

Countries vary widely in their ability to take action against NCDs. The DCP and GBD programmes have supported government leadership and their political will for a strong commitment to the health agenda by generating new knowledge and country level data to aid and assist decision-makers, especially those in the public sector, to realise the potential of affordable, effective interventions to rapidly improve the health and welfare of their populations.

WHO has furthered the agenda by providing national policymakers with a list of evidence-based "best buys" and other recommended interventions for the prevention and control of NCDs and to help reduce premature NCD deaths in the global south. These cover policy interventions that address the shared risk factors and clinical management interventions to reduce NCD morbidity and mortality. The growing burden of deaths from NCDs in low- and middle-income countries can be reduced through inexpensive population-based and clinical interventions. Fiscal policies are an especially promising and underused lever for reducing this burden (Jamison et al., 2013).

Governments should develop and implement a new economic paradigm for NCD action based on evidence that effective measures are investments in human capital and economic growth. They should increase the percentage of national budgets allocated to health, health promotion and essential public health functions; and within health to NCDs and mental health and disorders. This can be realised in part by implementing fiscal measures including raising taxes on tobacco and alcohol, and other unhealthy products like sugary drinks. With the support of tools developed by WHO, countries should conduct health-impact assessment and where possible full-cost accounting which factors in the true costs to societies of policies that have a bearing on NCDs.

The international community should assist governments by increasing financing and lending for the prevention and management of NCDs through bilateral and multilateral channels. This could include developing mechanisms to increase financing for NCD action, such as a global solidarity tobacco and alcohol contribution as a voluntary mechanism for member states for the prevention and treatment of NCDs; and a multi-donor fund to catalyse financing for the development of national NCD and mental health responses and policy coherence at country level. Other actions include integrating NCDs into human-capital and human development indices; and convening a health forum for investors to support action against NCDs.

Delivering NCD control interventions: investing in health systems strengthening

There are many fiscal measures and additional development assistance inflows that could be used by the government in the public sector to maximise health benefit and realise the potential of affordable, effective interventions to rapidly improve the health and mental well-being of their citizens and to prevent and control NCDs at the individual and population level. There is a set of health-improving strategies involving interventions to reduce modifiable risk factors and social determinants for NCDs and mental health through the creation of health-promoting environments for governments to invest in. In delivery terms, they can be considered as intersectoral and health-sector focussed.

Most intersectoral policies that impact health and mortality are fiscal levers, at the policy or legislative level or involve behavioural change or public education campaigns: they require less in the way of resources to implement compared to health-sector interventions; and are often one-off costs, explaining why so many are best buys and highly cost-effective. Significant political capital may be used when governments have to confront powerful vested interests and industry lobbying.

In contrast, health-sector interventions involve clinical management and biomedical prevention and require significant and sustained investment in health systems, human resources for health and quality service delivery for benefit to accrue equitably and to ensure that the poor, marginalised and underserved are included. This can make them less attractive as initial interventions and priorities for action when governments are developing their NCD implementation strategies. Intersectoral costs are largely without the health sector whereas health-sector interventions come from the health budget; almost all costs come from the public purse.

To be effective, clinical management interventions require strong, well-functioning health systems. In 2006, the Disease Control Priorities project examined cross-cutting issues crucial to the delivery of quality health services, including the organisation, financial support and capacity of health systems: their performance was subpar in most low- and middle-income countries. Strengthening health system performance requires action on many fronts and management levels that considers functions as well as associations between the system, its clients (patients) and their communities. Stewardship is important, particularly with community accountability and to ensure users have a voice and can influence priorities.

It is important to achieve a balance between vertical and horizontal modes of organisation and service delivery: disease-focussed verticalised efforts make the most sense in situations of weak capacity, poor governance and highly constrained resource availability. It is critical to strengthen the human resource base by reducing migration and improving recruitment and retention. Resources need to be directed equitably, and subsidies and incentives directed towards priority interventions (Laxminarayan et al., 2006).

Intersectoral policies and health-sector interventions to provide NCD services under an essential UHC umbrella were further examined in DCP-3 a decade later. Intersectoral policies fall into four broad categories: taxes and subsidies; regulations and related enforcement mechanisms; built environment; and information. They are managed and largely financed outside the health sector; when effectively implemented they will reduce disease risk and thus have a significant, if delayed impact on mortality, as it can take years for them to play out.

Interventions within the health sector that improve health outcomes will have a more immediate impact in reducing disease mortality. They were grouped into five platforms, defined as logistically related delivery platforms: population-based; community; health centre; first-level district hospital; and second-level referral or speciality hospital. In low- and middle-income countries, the modelled annual incremental costs of going from current service to full (80%) coverage of an essential high-priority health package was massive: over $100 billion in total, between $26–31 per person per year.

NCD Countdown 2030 is an independent global health collaboration to inform policies to reduce the burden of NCDs in low- and middle-income countries and to ensure accountability towards this. It recently updated costing data for delivering the most efficient high-priority NCD interventions. Reducing NCD mortality worldwide by one-third by 2030 would require annual incremental costs of US$140 billion in new spending: 39 million deaths could be averted; US$ 2.7 trillion in net economic benefit could be generated, benefits outweighing costs 19-to-1 (Watkins et al., 2022).

DCP-3 uniquely looks at incremental annual costs by healthcare level to show where investments need to be made. The breakdown of costs by platform is informative (Jamison et al., 2018):

- less than 1% for population-based intersectoral policy interventions
- 12–18% for community
- around 50–55% for health centres
- around 25% for first-level district hospitals
- between 6% and 9% for specialist referral hospitals

The majority of costs, around 70% are at the community or health centre level, clearly highlighting the need to make substantial new investment in person-centred PHC. This is strongly congruent with WHO and partner advocacy of the importance of PHC and a life course approach for NCD prevention and control. It is also in line with the Lancet Global Health Commission on financing PHC, with the proviso that it is important to finance both PHC and first- and second-level hospital care; and not favour PHC at the expense of hospital-level services (Hanson et al., 2022).

Fully 30% of incremental costs are for hospital services delivered at district second-level facilities or specialist referral hospitals; investment needs to be made into strengthening hospital services as well as into PHC. Guidelines for NCD clinical interventions at the PHC level have been produced: the HEARTS technical package for cardiovascular disease management in PHC (World Health Organization (WHO), 2018b); the WHO PEN package of essential NCD interventions for PHC (World Health Organization (WHO), 2020). Users require significant knowledge, core clinical management skills and access to laboratory services. Referral pathways to second-level hospital care are widely recommended, and there is a requirement for a very well-stocked pharmacy more likely to be found at hospital than at the PHC or community level.

8 The NCDs: increasingly important, still neglected and in crisis

Inadequate progress in addressing the NCD epidemic in the global south

There are very good data and high recognition that the burden of disease in the global south is rapidly shifting towards chronic non-communicable diseases (NCDs). It is clear what needs to be done to address the NCD epidemic: we know how they can be prevented and how they can be managed. Cost-effective interventions exist and much has been written on what to do to prevent or manage NCDs in all their complexity, accepting that cost-effectiveness data indicate what a reasonably well-functioning health system can achieve. The NCDs have been discussed at the UN in three high-level meetings (HLMs) and appear prominently in the UN 2030 Agenda for Sustainable Development. An ambitious sustainable development goal (SDG) target, to reduce NCD mortality by one-third by 2030, has been widely adopted by countries in the global south. Despite all this, limited progress has been made, and the NCDs remain neglected and in crisis.

In 2018, the NCD countdown 2030 collaboration emphasised that NCD mortality is higher in low- and middle-income countries, and in high-income countries in people with lower socio-economic status, making NCDs an important obstacle to reducing global and national health inequalities. The group noted that the risks of dying from NCDs were particularly high in sub-Saharan Africa and for men in Central Asia and Eastern Europe. Mortality has stagnated or even increased since 2010 in 10% of countries; those on track to achieving the SDG mortality target are mostly high-income countries. Substantial reduction of NCD mortality requires policies to be implemented to reduce tobacco and alcohol use and control blood pressure; and provide equitable access to efficacious and high-quality preventative and curative care for acute and chronic NCDs (Bennett et al., 2018).

The final 2019 report of the WHO Independent Commission on NCDs "Its Time to Walk the Talk" highlighted that progress against NCDs and mental health conditions must be greatly accelerated if targets are to be achieved and the

DOI: 10.4324/9781003505693-11

2030 agenda is to succeed. Countries face significant challenges in implementing the ambitious commitments they have made. The majority have not fulfilled their commitment to complement policy, legislative and regulatory measures by strengthening health literacy through education; nor have they implemented population-wide and targeted social media campaigns that provide information to the public about risk factors for NCDs.

Countries have yet to establish national multisectoral or transparent accountability mechanisms and are still to implement whole-of-government and whole-of-society approaches for health in all policies. Limited progress has been made in securing effective and meaningful commitments and actions from the private sector. Few have fulfilled commitments to implement policy, legislative and regulatory mechanisms aimed at minimising the impact of the main NCD risk factors. Funding for NCDs and mental health falls far behind what is required: the commission recommended that higher percentages of national budgets are allocated to health, and that within health a higher proportion is allocated to NCDs and mental health, financed partly through higher taxes on tobacco and alcohol (World Health Organization (WHO), 2019b).

Effectively tackling NCDs and tracking progress requires a detailed understanding of the current status and progress being made at country level, and information about where gaps and blocks may be developing. WHO in the NCD progress monitor regularly reports against a set of ten agreed progress monitoring indicators intended to show the progress achieved in countries in the implementation of selected national commitments that span the prevention and control of NCDs: some indicators have multiple components making 19 activities, policies and plans for reporting against at the state level. Most relate to the implementation of intersectoral policies; only two focus on health sector and clinical disease management interventions (Table 8.1).

Longitudinal analysis of global policy data from 2014 to 2021, covering 194 countries and reported in four NCD progress monitor reports showed that over the period, wide geographical variation has persisted: policy implementation is lowest in the African region, and highest in rich high-income countries. NCD policy implementation has stagnated from 2019 to 2021: progress in the implementation of some policies was offset by the reduced implementation of others, including those relating to physical activity, national NCD planning and consumption patterns of unhealthy commodities, such as tobacco, alcohol and unhealthy foods and sugary soft drinks. One particular issue identified with the inadequate action taken on alcohol, food and tobacco use was the absence of safeguards against corporate financial influence over policy-making (Allen et al., 2023).

The SARS-CoV-2 pandemic has severely disrupted health systems, interrupted and set back efforts to protect people and populations from NCDs: people with NCDs are also at increased risk of severe COVID-19 disease or death. An online survey of front-line healthcare workers in primary care from nine

Table 8.1 The ten NCD progress monitoring indicators for Member State activities

Member State NCD control activities	➢ Relevant progress monitoring indicators
Consider developing national multisectoral policies and plans to achieve national targets by 2025	1: Member State has set time-bound national targets based on WHO Guidance 2: Member State has a functioning system for generating reliable cause-specific mortality data on a routine basis 3: Member State has a STEPS survey or a comprehensive health examination survey every five years 4: Member State has an operational multisectoral national strategy/action plan that integrates the major NCDs and their shared risk factors
Reduce risk factors for NCDs, building on guidance set out in the WHO Global NCD Action Plan	5: Member State has implemented the five demand-reduction measures for Tobacco control in the WHO FCTC at the highest level of achievement 6: Member State has implemented as appropriate according to national circumstances three measures to reduce the harmful use of alcohol 7: Member State has implemented four measures to reduce unhealthy diet: reduce salt intake; limit saturated and trans fatty acids in food; implement the international code of marketing of breast-milk substitutes; control the marketing of food and non-alcoholic beverages to children 8: Member State has implemented at least one recent national public awareness and motivational communication for physical activity
Strengthen health systems to address NCDs through people-centred primary health care and universal health coverage, building on guidance set out in the WHO Global NCD Action Plan	9: Member State has evidence-based national guidelines/protocols/standards for the management of major NCDs through a primary care approach approved by government or competent authorities 10: Member State has provision of drug therapy including glycaemic control and counselling for eligible persons at high risk to prevent heart attacks and stroke with emphasis on the primary care level

low- and middle-income countries found that patient care had been adversely impacted by public health measures imposed, which particularly impacted on continuity of care. Almost all reported a deterioration in the mental health of their patients (Bullen et al., 2021).

The most recent 2022 WHO NCD Progress Monitor further highlighted limited progress and missed opportunities. It confirmed that COVID-19 has severely disrupted health systems and set back efforts to protect people and populations from NCDs. While over 120 Member States have an operational multisector national strategy or action plan for NCDs and 77 countries have fully achieved more indicators in 2022 compared with 2020, more than 50 have lost ground, achieving fewer indicators than in 2020. Although more countries are running campaigns to reduce tobacco use and develop clinical guidelines, there have been major declines in physical activity awareness campaigns, the development of integrated NCD plans and NCD surveillance. Premature mortality has increased in more than 20 mostly low- and middle-income countries. It seems that simple and effective interventions are not being adopted widely enough around the world to impact the NCD pandemic and reduce morbidity and mortality (World Health Organization (WHO), 2022b).

To date, there has been relatively little evaluation of health sector-focussed interventions. One study looking at the HEARTS technical package for CVD risk assessment and management, also promoted in WHO PENS, using representative data from 40 low- and middle-income countries found very low use of statins, antihypertensives and aspirin for either the primary or secondary prevention of CVD in eligible patients (Zhu et al., 2023). This is despite the strong and accumulating evidence of the value of the "polypill", the fixed-dose combination medicine comprised of blood-pressure-lowering medication with a statin to reduce cholesterol, with or without aspirin, in substantially reducing cardiovascular disease and death in the global south (Joseph et al., 2021).

Resources are not matching the size and scale of the NCD crisis

Little can be done without appropriate funding: insufficient financial resources have been raised to make much of an impact on the NCD crisis, despite being very high up on the global policy agenda and having been discussed in the United Nations in several HLMs. Like other health-related topics that have been discussed at the United Nations (HIV/AIDS; antimicrobial resistance; TB; universal health coverage (UHC)) both national commitments and international political commitments have increased. However, financing for prevention and control of NCDs has been stagnant at the domestic level and while international funding has increased, it has been insufficient to really make a difference. As a result, the outcome of the HLM meetings have had limited impact on the global NCD crisis. In fact, only for HIV/AIDS has discussion at the UN had any strong outcome on financing the global health challenge been achieved (Rodi et al., 2022).

The WHO global coordinating mechanism on NCDs convened a working group to explore financing for NCDs with an emphasis on low- and middle-income countries. It noted in 2016 that global funding is insufficient to attain the nine targets of the WHO global action plan on NCDs. The share of development assistance for health (DAH) dedicated to NCDs has remained at 1–2% of the total since 2000. The primacy of domestic funding, dominated by out-of-pocket (OOP) payments, can be complimented by additional revenue from taxation, loans, the private sector and innovative financing mechanisms though these will take time to be generated. In the interim there is a clear role for development assistance to bridge the gap. In the long-term countries will hopefully assume financial responsibility for preventing and controlling NCDs (Allen, 2017).

An analysis of the policy and funding priorities of global actors noted that they increasingly recognised the growing threat of NCDs and their drivers. However, while they provided over 80% of development assistance committed to NCDs in low- and middle-income countries, NCDs are still under-prioritised; policy priorities and funding allocations need to better align to address the NCD epidemic (Jailobaeva et al., 2021).

In 2022, NCD Countdown 2030 emphasised that substantial reduction of NCD mortality requires policies that reduce tobacco and alcohol use and blood pressure as well as support equitable access to efficacious and high-quality preventative and curative care; countries were off track in delivery with considerable implementation constraints, especially from COVID-19-related health system disruptions. Looking forward to help countries get back on track, a framework for NCD investment was proposed, centred around a model package of 21 interventions that are feasible to implement and can form the backbone of national NCD strategies, with countries choosing what is most suitable to their situation.

Implementing the most efficient package of interventions in each world region would require on average an additional US$ 18 billion annually: these costs would comprise around 20% of national health budgets, a considerable increase for low- and middle-income countries. Some domestic funding could come from higher taxes on tobacco and alcohol; additional resources would almost certainly have to come from development assistance (Watkins et al., 2022).

It remains unclear exactly how sufficient additional resources will be raised and how the profound changes in health financing are to come about to appropriately strengthen health systems in the global south to deliver on the NCD agenda. A decade ago, it was evident that health systems in low- and middle-income countries were not functioning effectively enough to make progress on the NCD agenda and achieve universal coverage for healthcare. Evidence on the deficiencies of healthcare systems and their financing far exceeds evidence on remedies to improve healthcare. There is a lack of financial support for those who need healthcare: on average, almost 50% of healthcare financing in low-income countries comes from OOP payments.

It is commonly accepted that the poorest people require complete subsidisation for healthcare costs from general taxation, with donors also contributing through pro-poor support schemes. Financial incentives may work in some situations, and privatisation of parts of service delivery may also work. An approach that works well in one country may work less well in another; and not all approaches are equally acceptable to all governments or their multiple constituencies. Healthcare systems are complex social constructs: their strengthening must be seen as a long-term development process (Mills, 2014).

The only time that there has been a significant, sustained upturn in healthcare funding since 1990 has been during what has been called the glory years for global health spending, the decade from 2000 to 2009 when DAH from both bilateral and multilateral funding sources increased at a staggering 11.3% per year (Nugent, 2016). DAH makes up around half of the health budgets in low-income countries. Over the period just 1.2% of all DAH went to fund the NCD agenda whereas the vast bulk went to support the three health goals in the millenium development goals (MDG): MDG 4, a two-thirds reduction in under-5 mortality; MDG 5, a reduction of maternal mortality by three-quarters; and MDG 6, a reversal of the spread of HIV/AIDS, malaria, tuberculosis and other major infectious diseases. This was why the global health community was so keen to get the NCDs prominently included in the SDGs. Unfortunately, DAH has flatlined since then for all disease control priorities, communicable and non-communicable alike (Dieleman et al., 2016).

As already noted, primary healthcare (PHC) has a critical role in the NCD agenda: it puts people at the centre, is recognised as a key component of all high-performing health systems and is the best platform for providing basic health interventions equitably. The Lancet Global Health Commission on financing PHC recently reported that in most low- and middle-income countries, PHC does not meet the needs of the people who should be at its centre. Public funding is insufficient, access to services remains inequitable, and patients often have to pay OOP to use them.

A vicious cycle has undermined PHC: underfunded services that are unreliable and of poor quality are bypassed by sick people in favour of higher-level specialist care. Fundamentally shifting a health system's priorities away from specialist- and hospital-based services and towards PHC involves political choices and creates numerous political and service delivery challenges. Across the global south, countries spend far too little on PHC to provide equitable access to essential services. The focus needs to be on strengthening financing for PHC; all countries need to both invest more and invest better (Hanson et al., 2022).

Scrutinising why progress on the NCD agenda has been slow and inadequate

Why has such limited progress been made when so much time and effort has been spent describing the NCD crisis across the global south, highlighting that they are a neglected development issue with a very strong case for urgent global action; noting the critically important linkages with both the PHC and UHC agendas; and despite the growing consensus on priority actions and best buy interventions to address the NCD epidemic? Several problems seem to exist; the list below is not exhaustive and others may well be contributing.

First, there is the nebulous NCD construct: even when the agenda has been simplified down to the five-by-five approach, the groups actually break down to multiple individual diseases; and the shared risk factors present a heterogeneous set of policy actions and structural interventions. The brand has limited public recognition and generates little awareness about the importance of the NCD agenda and the implementation crisis with inadequate action to control the NCDs effectively.

It has already been pointed out that there is little that can be done now with the construct, though more should be done to overcome some of the inconsistencies and break down the false dichotomies and seemingly competing priorities: transmissible or non-communicable, prevention or care and treatment. A broader concept like disease control priorities which avoids these problems has also failed to generate public recognition and much action. This may have been because DCP tended to overemphasise the economic evaluation of health interventions over other important factors including health equity and the right to health (Rumbold et al., 2017).

Second, there are the composite goals and targets: SDG Global Goal 3 "good health and wellbeing" is all-encompassing, lacks punch and is rather anodyne. Outcome target 3.4 is to reduce by one-third premature mortality from NCDs through prevention and treatment by 2030 and to promote mental health and well-being: being a composite, the all-NCD mortality rate target lacks specificity and does not readily relate to the recognised diseases like heart attacks or diabetes that voters and taxpayers know and care about, with resonance only to those with an understanding of global public health. The suicide rate means little except to health professionals. Both are modelled estimates.

While a rate can be reported on at global and country level, shifting an estimate up or down has limited meaning to the general public at the individual and community level particularly when campaigns on health literacy have stalled: it really does not and cannot lead to any sense of urgency around the need for funds and action. A 2030 deadline favours health sector interventions which can relatively quickly impact morbidity and mortality rather than policy interventions which can take decades to show results on health: paradoxically the policy interventions are favoured over clinical management. The means of achieving

SDG 3 targets lack specificity: reducing alcohol use and air pollution are rather nebulous in the absence of targeted social media campaigns; implementing the FCTC, investing more in research and universal access to medicines and vaccines, and increasing health financing and health workforce density seem remote to the poorly understood NCD agenda.

Third, there is the lack of civil society engagement and NCD activism that is critical to push for more domestic funding for health, better targeted to priority diseases that the public cares about, suffers from and want access to quality treatment and care. With a fuzzy construct, indistinct goals and a general lack of health literacy and knowledge about NCD risk factors, it may be too much to expect civil society activists or pressure groups to form and rally vocally around the obesity epidemic, air pollution, premature deaths from smoking or inequitable CVD outcomes widening between rich countries and the global south; and then advocate for policy, legislative and regulatory measures for whole-of-government and whole-of-society approaches for NCD prevention and control.

Mental health challenges are orphan issues in the global north and south alike. Strong civil society lobbying is also important to influence voters and taxpayers to press for increased bilateral and multilateral DAH for health in general, with appropriate allocations for covering the NCD agenda; and to loudly call for social justice and health equity. Without it, the silence is deafening; it is hardly surprising that funding has remained so far off track.

Fourth, many years into the NCD crisis, there is unfortunately little concrete and tangible progress to report back to give donors and politicians the confidence to upscale investment in NCD prevention and control and to establish national multisectoral and transparent accountability mechanisms. Without success stories to refer to, particularly in the care and treatment area the general public is most interested in and concerned about, it is not clear what will drive the political process and result in more appropriate and equitable resource allocation for NCD control.

Reducing risk by managing consumption through increasing taxes on tobacco and alcohol may well be a best buy and can potentially generate revenue for NCD control, but fiscal measures will be unpopular and take years to have a measurable health impact. Behaviour change through mass media campaigns for reducing salt or increasing physical activity will have prevention benefit but is relatively invisible in its downstream health impacts to community. There has been limited input into more tangible biomedical prevention interventions, such as rolling out drug therapy for CVD and diabetes management; or for stroke management, rehabilitation and care for diabetic complications. Vaccination campaigns to prevent HPV or HBV will only have an impact on cervical or liver cancer many years down the line; and is only appreciated with relatively high levels of health literacy.

Fifth, the impact of the SARS-CoV-2/COVID-19 pandemic has been significant across the global south. It has disrupted health systems and set back efforts to protect people and populations from NCDs. People living with NCDs are at increased risk of severe COVID-19 disease or death: health staff have been moved over to deal with COVID-19 clinical services and continuity of NCD care has been disrupted by public health measures implemented to contain the pandemic. As the COVID-19 PHEIC has ended, it is hoped that health services in low- and middle-income countries will quickly recover and resources will be re-prioritised back to disease-specific control programmes, including the NCDs and mental health. But they will remain inadequate as pandemic preparedness takes precedence.

Finally, there are the perennial challenges with generating more funding for healthcare in general, and in particular allocating more resources to primary healthcare. Funding is political as the Lancet Commission on financing PHC emphasised. But suggesting that health funds are diverted from specialist-based and hospital-based care to PHC implies healthcare financing is a zero-sum game. Rather the issue is to improve the quality of care at both primary and secondary levels which requires more resources for health staff and preventive and curative services. It must not be either primary care or hospital care: this is another false dichotomy. It has to be both, something the general public recognise and appreciate, particularly when there is general acceptance that the poorest people require complete subsidisation for healthcare costs from general taxation. Quality care is costly but has to be paid for along with delivering on the best buy policies to prevent NCDs.

What can be done or done differently to move the NCD agenda forward

Identifying some of the reasons for such slow progress on the NCD agenda to date leads on to a discussion about what can be done now or done differently with the current paradigm to drive action at country level to address the NCD crisis. Several lessons from the successes that HIV/AIDS control programmes have had in the global south are relevant to inform this discussion.

One key lesson from HIV/AIDS is that a prevention only approach is insufficient and has very limited community buy-in. Budget holders and politicians are attracted to best buys if almost all are at the policy level, with limited health system implementation costs; and the potential to generate revenue if fiscal measures are also enacted. But communities need and expect more for sick individuals for whom prevention has failed and policy has been introduced too late to stop disease and premature death: treatment and clinical care is needed. If not available in the public sector, this will be paid for OOP if the household can afford the costs imposed by an NCD, either for obtaining medical care, or from the lost income associated with being ill and unable to work.

Illness imposes a very heavy burden on households; poor households are the most financially affected when they seek care (Kankeu et al., 2013). National multisectoral and transparent accountability mechanisms for the implementation of whole-of-government and whole-of-society approaches for health in all policies are important but insufficient. Tangible improvements are needed in biomedical prevention, diagnosis, care and treatment to protect the poorest households. Intersectoral policies, legislation and regulatory measures on tobacco, alcohol, sodium, healthy food, exercise by themselves are not enough and will not generate civil society engagement; policy must be accompanied by practice in NCD management and care.

HIV/AIDS showed the importance of activists and pressure groups to promote equitable access to ART and close the treatment gap, and then universal access to biomedical prevention. Civil society engagement is limited with poor health literacy on the NCDs particularly when much of the agenda is policies for healthy living or to prevent NCDs rather than how to treat them. And when there is such a limited understanding of the nebulous NCD construct.

It does not have to be so: one way to short-circuit this is to focus on global NCD treatment targets 8 and 9; and foster and create community demand for health services action and delivery. Screening for cardiac risk factors will identify those who need essential medicines to lower cholesterol and blood pressure and to achieve control of blood sugar: target 8 is that at least 50% receive drug therapy. Campaigns for health literacy should focus on increasing community understanding about affordable basic technologies and essential medicines to screen and treat NCDs in the public sector: target 9 is 80% availability in public and private facilities (World Health Organization (WHO), 2013).

The HIV/AIDS response showed the centrality and importance of people living with HIV/AIDS as active and vocal advocates for care and treatment that they knew they would need, sometimes when they were sick, immediately: PLHA were very strong advocates for person-centred AIDS care. Attempts have been made to create an active community of people living with NCDs (PLWNCD) in the post-Covid world, aiming to build back better and to optimise the relevance of NCD and mental health priorities, policies and practices (World Health Organization (WHO), 2021b). More should be done: such a community of practice is well placed to articulate for person-centred care that has to involve treatment and be delivered at the primary care level and also involve district hospitals.

Chronic NCDs, like HIV/AIDS, are complex to treat at the primary care level; and are incurable requiring lifelong clinical care that seems challenging to sustain at the population-level. Guidelines for care at the PHC level exist, such as the HEARTS technical package for cardiovascular disease management or the WHO PEN package of essential NCD interventions for primary healthcare; but they are really quite complex to use, assume access to well-stocked pharmacies and referral to specialist hospitals.

One progress monitoring indicator is the approval of evidence-based guidelines, protocols and standards for the management of major NCDs through a primary care approach recognised and approved by government or a competent authorities. The experience of HIV/AIDS programmes is that such complex guidelines need to be simplified and standardised by following a public health approach so they can be rolled out at PHC level and integrated with specialist second-level services (Gilks et al., 2006).

It is vital to build an NCD-ready workforce, just as it was to build an HIV/AIDS-ready workforce to deliver biomedical HIV prevention and AIDS care and treatment through targeted investments in health systems strengthening and service delivery. Having sufficient human resources for health who are skilled and competent in NCD prevention and treatment is an absolute minimal requirement for delivering on the NCD agenda. The importance of UHC and PHC in shaping more effective health systems to deliver services for the prevention and control of NCDs was made in the 2023 extension of the NCD global action plan looking forward to 2030 (World Health Organization (WHO), 2023a).

WHO held a meeting in June 2021 on building an NCD-ready workforce with support from the UHC partnership which helps leverage WHO's technical expertise in advancing UHC with a primary care approach. The strategic roundtable explored key activities needed to prompt urgent action on multiple fronts to meet the global demand for health workers to deliver NCD care through population-based planning and policy-making and to build capacities of existing and future health and multisectoral workers in critical competencies needed for NCD prevention and care. It recognised the need to empower communities as providers of NCD care to lessen the burden on health services, and to engage workers and PLWNCD as champion providers of NCD care (World Health Organization (WHO), 2023b).

Finally, it is important to embrace and accept the scope for NCD action is widening with progressive universalism, a pathway to UHC that particularly focusses on social justice and pro-poor policies because the poor are disproportionately impacted by ill health. Stronger health systems are needed for the delivery of core NCD prevention and control; and beyond that to UHC. A wider set of activities and a stronger health system that is able to deliver quality and effective care requires significant new funding, domestically and through DAH. AIDS activists in the global north and south pressurised politicians everywhere on the right to health, to do more on treatment equity and to exceptionally allocate more resources to a clear agenda for universal access to ART. Somehow a movement for social justice and NCD health and treatment has to be fashioned by civil society and PLWNCD. There is a right to health which includes NCD services; without more funding for the health sector, the NCD agenda will never be delivered on.

9   A public health approach to scale up NCD control interventions

A new paradigm for NCD prevention and control in the global south

Some tweaks can be made to the way non-communicable diseases (NCDs) are currently conceptualised and approached, guided by lessons learned from HIV/AIDS control programmes; but they are unlikely to generate a step change in intersectoral policy implementation or a surge in health system strengthening to sharply impact NCD prevention and control in low- and middle-income countries. It is unlikely that there will be any significant upturn in resources either from domestic or international sources anytime soon. On the current trajectory, it seems inevitable that sustainable development goal (SDG) target 3.4, to reduce premature NCD mortality by one-third by 2030, will not be achieved.

A new paradigm for NCD prevention and control in the global south is now needed. The key is to strongly pivot to the health sector for the rapid implementation of health-improving treatment strategies; and to expand health services that address the patient perspective and provide access to quality clinical services for prevention or care to deal with the burden of ill-health and premature death from NCDs on the individual, their household and community.

Governments will need to find substantial new funds for health system and services improvement and allocate additional public finances to meet social goals of improving population health and reducing the financial risks of ill-health. Development assistance will also need to be stepped up. This seems the only feasible way that premature NCD mortality can be quickly impacted and significantly reduced by 2030.

A strong pivot to the health sector for AIDS treatment to address sick patient needs has worked very well in low- and middle-income countries: exceptionally supported vertical HIV/AIDS programmes provide quality antiretroviral therapy (ART) services for free in the public sector. As discussed in the first section, there are many reasons for this: vocal activism for an exceptional response; an unprecedented political commitment to closing the treatment gap; the creation of new bilateral and multilateral funding mechanisms; clear and simple goals and

DOI: 10.4324/9781003505693-12

targets; a conceptually radical WHO public health approach to care and treatment; and clear guidelines for public sector implementation of treatment then biomedical prevention. Global ART coverage exceeds 75% and is still rising.

Initially ART was a specialist-led hospital-based service: the public health approach was rolled out; ART was simplified and standardised; clinical services were strengthened; and delivery massively scaled up. Treatment initiation and long-term treatment support was increasingly provided at the primary care level and involved first-level hospitals and district management teams decongesting specialist hospitals.

Task-shifting supports primary healthcare (PHC) treatment and facilitates person-centred care but does not obviate the need for hospital referral when serious clinical problems develop. Sustaining universal access to ART long-term is impossible without quality care at the PHC level that is accessible to all; and is the textbook example of the importance of PHC in the effective delivery of person-centred care at the community level.

Free ART is pro-poor, reducing the financial burden of ill-health for the person living with HIV, and the risk of catastrophic health expenditure on their household. As such, successful HIV/AIDS control programmes can be considered a successful if circumscribed textbook example of how universal health coverage (UHC) can be achieved in communities of people living with HIV, albeit within a vertical programme. It is also from the DCP-3 perspective a model example of essential universal health coverage that successfully is addressing a major single disease control priority.

Building a public health approach for NCDs: the pivot to health systems and services

A paradigm shift in how NCD control is conceptualised and approached is urgently needed to impact significantly chronic disease morbidity and premature mortality in the global south. This involves a major pivot to the provision of health-improving clinical interventions by a strengthened health system that can deliver effective quality treatment for disease management and linked biomedical prevention; and that is actively person-centred and patient-focussed.

A fairly prescriptive way to do this can be mapped out, building on existing management protocols and based on the core tenets of the WHO public health approach to ART (Gilks et al., 2006). This approach has successfully underpinned HIV/AIDS control in the global south such that HIV is now endemic rather than epidemic in most communities; and the end of AIDS by 2030 is regarded as feasible in many jurisdictions (Assefa & Gilks, 2020).

The key conceptual shift was the move from individual, physician-led therapy to a population-based public health approach, recognised as the only way to rapidly and equitably make ART accessible through the public health system to the millions in need across the global south. The public health approach was person and patient-centred: it emphasised the centrality of delivering ART across the life-course; and clarified how clinical teams in primary care and second-level facilities were effectively enabled to deliver ART equitably to all in need in resource-constrained setting.

Screening and diagnosis: The first step is to provide simple diagnostic testing and screening for the major chronic NCDs at the primary care level with results available as soon as possible so the next steps can be discussed with the client and planned with the clinical team. The next steps vary: with a negative test or screening result below an initiation threshold, appropriate health promotion information for diet, smoking, exercise and so on can be given with a short explanation of why this helps prevents downstream clinical problems and premature death; with a positive screening result above threshold, the appropriate biomedical prevention intervention should be commenced accompanied by relevant health promotion information; with a positive diagnostic test result, appropriate treatment should be started with a specialist referral if indicated.

For most NCDs, screening and diagnostic testing involve simple on-the-spot measurements: blood pressure (BP) using an inflatable arm cuff; electrocardiograph (ECG) heart trace; height and weight to assess body-mass index (BMI) and obesity; spirometry breath test for airway obstruction and respiratory function. For diabetes, this will involve a point-of-care (POC) finger-prick blood sugar test using a hand-held analyser. POC test strips are available to assess cholesterol and other blood lipid levels but need a bench-top analyser. Simple POC diagnostic tests are available for a wide variety of chronic infections, including HIV, Hepatitis B and C.

Some test results may need confirmation or indicate further blood tests and investigations. Basic radiography should be available in district or first-level hospitals and can help assess cardiovascular status, diagnose TB or lung cancer in one clinical session. Cancer screening involves recognition of common cancer signs and symptoms and urgent referral to a second-level facility; diagnosis is not generally feasible at the PHC level.

From the client or patient's perspective, differentiating biobehavioural prevention interventions like smoking cessation, avoiding alcohol, promoting healthy diets and physical activity from biomedical prevention interventions that use medicines to reduce blood pressure or blood glucose, manage COPD airflow obstruction or replace nicotine; or vaccination to prevent cancer make no sense. Following a positive result, the individual needs access to a continuum of interventions that can treat or prevent NCDs; community needs health-improving policies to be enacted, support for self-care and ready access to screening and diagnostic services at the primary care level.

From the health system perspective it is important to differentiate fiscal and policy interventions which are without the remit of health from the clinical interventions that health services need to provide once the need for biomedical prevention or disease management has been identified through screening and diagnostic testing. NCD screening is the entry point to biomedical prevention, as NCD testing is to treatment. Quality services are costly and can be complex to provide across the continuum when there are several major chronic diseases and many different treatments.

If quality clinical services cannot be delivered there is little point in providing NCD screening and diagnosis. The bottom line is that once a test has identified the need to intervene, the appropriate treatment needs to be accessible and made available. Without biomedical prevention or care and treatment, there will be little individual interest in, or uptake of screening or diagnostic testing in primary care; community will not respond or engage with NCD screening campaigns; resources invested in screening will largely be wasted.

Standardised treatments and simple formularies: The essence of the WHO public health approach as initially developed for ART was the standardisation of treatment regimens and the simplification of drug formularies that would support equitable access, facilitate rapid scale-up and allow effective quality delivery. It aimed to set global treatment standards that were applicable to all in need of life-saving therapy regardless of location.

The most important component was to standardise ART around first then second-line treatment regimens for population-wide delivery, in contrast to the initial regimen a specialist physician would prescribe for their patient, subsequently changing ARVs according to response. A choice was made to simplify formularies around the agreed ART regimens so that there was just one main first-line combination regimen made available through public sector health facilities; and one second-line regimen when first-line therapy was failing. A pragmatic evidence-informed decision was made as to which medicines to recommend for first-line ART and which to reserve for second-line.

There are two NCD packages which make standardised recommendations on medicines for primary and secondary biomedical prevention or disease management at the PHC level: the HEARTS technical package for cardiovascular disease management (World Health Organization (WHO), 2018b); and the WHO PEN package of essential NCDs interventions (World Health Organization (WHO), 2020) which incorporates HEARTS protocols and has updated protocols for diabetes, chronic respiratory diseases (CRDs) and early cancer diagnosis.

Both HEARTS and PEN are intended for use by policymakers and programme managers at different levels within national Ministries of Health who can influence NCD primary care delivery, rather than end-users. They support the development of national strategies, policies and plans related to service delivery; help set national targets, guide progress monitoring and reporting; and assist in training. All modules and protocol recommendations are expected to require adaptation at country level.

- *Cardiovascular disease management*: The pharmacological protocols for treating raised BP note there are four main classes of antihypertensive medicines: complex recommendations are made for first and second-line options, depending on whether there is underlying heart disease or stroke. Medicines can also be used in some situations in combination. Referral to a specialist is recommended if blood pressure cannot be controlled despite second-line therapy and if the patient has been fully adherent and taken their medication as prescribed. Lifestyle management is recommended for all patients. Despite promotion of risk-based CVD management with country-specific risk charts that include blood cholesterol levels, there is a current gap with no pharmacological protocols yet developed for the choice and use of lipid lowering statin medicines to manage elevated cholesterol; or for the polypill, a combination medicine of an aspirin, a statin and an ACE inhibitor to lower BP for both primary and secondary prevention of cardiovascular disease (Rodgers & Smith, 2023).

• *Diabetes management*: The pharmacological protocols for treating diabetes note that there are two main classes of oral medicines as well as injectable insulin which can be deployed to reduce blood sugar; and make recommendations for first-line, second-line and third-line treatment. However, the choice of which medicine to use first depends on blood glucose levels; and third-line insulin injections will only be available at hospital level. Referral for specialist management is recommended when blood sugar control has not been achieved after 2–3 months. Lifestyle management is recommended for all patients.

• *Chronic respiratory diseases*: The pharmacological protocols for CRDs cover exacerbations of asthma and management of COPD; children are included in the asthma section. Severity is assessed to guide which medicines are recommended for use and whether antibiotics are indicated. These are simpler because there are a limited set of medicines which are effective in the management of CRD. There are no pathways for specialist hospital referral. Lifestyle management is recommended for all patients.

• *Cancer early diagnosis*: Cancer symptoms can be non-specific and early diagnosis of cervical cancer or breast cancer often relies on identifying "red flag" signs and symptoms. If these are identified, then urgent referral to specialist hospital services is indicated to initiate appropriate treatment. There are no pharmacological protocols for cancer treatment at the primary care level. Lifestyle management is recommended for all patients as is widescale vaccination for HBV and HPV prevention.

The focus in these packages is on PHC delivery of specific NCD clinical management interventions. As they stand, many of the recommendations are more relevant for physician-led decision-making; and are excessively complex for non-physicians to use at primary care level to support population-wide NCD care and treatment. The extensive list of recommended first-, second- and third-line treatments need significant simplification to produce formularies better suited to a community pharmacy with limited stocks of essential medicines.

The packages will be difficult to adapt to suit country realities and be simplified down to formularies that support equitable population access in resource-constrained settings. Many countries only have a limited cadre of experienced physicians with significant expertise in reviewing standard treatment approaches who can readily simplify formularies according to reality; and accept that their health services often do not have the capacity at PHC or referral hospital level to be able to effectively implement complex treatment pathways using multiple regimens based on individual clinical presentation and response.

More work is urgently needed to further standardise approaches and simplify formularies for front-line clinicians to use. WHO and partners must take bold, strong technical leadership to develop a public health approach to NCDs. Expert groups will need to be convened, tasked to more rigorously develop standardised treatments and simpler formularies; and then work with countries to support direct implementation or regional adaptations based on local context. Difficult technical choices will have to be made based on practicality and country reality rather than perfection, focussing strongly on what can be delivered at primary care level and district hospital level.

Simplified clinical decision-making and standardised monitoring: As the process for standardising treatments and simplifying formularies starts, consideration can be given to the clinical decision-making steps that are involved in the effective delivery of NCD interventions at primary care and district hospital levels by a wide cadre of different healthcare workers; and that recognise the limited capacity and infrastructure that will exist as NCD care and treatment scales up as additional funds and resources are provided.

One of the critical conceptual developments in the public health approach to ART was removing the decision taken by a physician on which medicines to prescribe for initial and subsequent treatment. This is not needed in public health sector ART because just one main first-line and one second-line option is provided, usually for free. The main clinical decisions instead involve the four S's: when to start first-line, when to substitute with an alternate first-line medicine, when to switch to second-line with first-line failure, and when to stop for futility and move to end-of-life palliative care.

This simple paradigm attracted much criticism, as specialist physicians and experts widely believed that one size could not fit all. But it proved remarkably robust and enabled rapid equitable ART scale-up across the global south. The approach can readily be applied and used for NCD management:

- *When to start* an intervention after screening for high BP, diabetes or COPD has been dealt with in HEARTS and WHO PEN packages by adopting and using internationally agreed thresholds for initiating clinical treatment, with relevant lifestyle management and health promotion information given to all. These need little or no modification as they are global consensus norms.

- *When to substitute* one first-line medicine for another within the same class because of intolerance or toxicity to preserve downstream options may not exist when there is only one first-line medicine. In ART when to substitute arises with severe drug toxicity or drug-drug interactions with treatment for comorbidities. Medicines for most chronic NCDs are generally well tolerated but toxicity will still occur as will drug-drug interactions. Some can be easily recognised and managed at PHC level; most will require referral for diagnosis and specialist management. It may be necessary to substitute with a new class of medicine.
- *When to switch* to second-line treatment for poor initial or waning response to first-line treatment rests on three issues: whether there is a clear binary first then second-line treatment option, as with blood pressure control and diabetes but not with CRDs; how failure or non-response is defined and assessed, which will usually be by continuing to measure the screening value like blood pressure or blood sugar; and what the second or third-line option is, and whether it is only available at hospital level.
- *When to stop* for futility and move to end-of-life care is important but mainly a consideration in cancer care; when there is intractable and refractory heart failure; or in chronic kidney disease and other pernicious complications of diabetes management. The PEN package of essential NCD interventions for PHC has guidance material for palliative care.

Clinical decisions for NCD medicine use could be further simplified down to just three steps: when to start, when to change (amalgamating substitution and switching) and when to stop.

ART is started following a positive HIV test. One programmatic issue is the need for a different viral load test to monitor treatment response that is not generally available in primary care. This will not be a problem that impacts standardised monitoring of NCD interventions as the same test that is used for screening or diagnosis is used for monitoring the clinical response. Thresholds to trigger when to switch NCD treatment to second-line are widely agreed on.

Simple standard implementation guidelines: Once a simplified and standardised set of treatments for NCD prevention and management have been developed with consensus on simplified clinical decision-making and standardised monitoring, it becomes straightforward to generate a set of complimentary packages for managing major NCDs in resource-constrained settings. This should be done under the auspices and technical leadership of WHO, with support and inputs from experts, key partners and stakeholders, including PLWNCD groups and community; and with countries fully engaged and involved at all steps of the process.

Using a standard template for each NCD, it is an easy next step to integrate these together into a simple easy to use standard treatment guideline for a public health approach for scaling up NCD interventions in resource-limited settings, exactly as was done for HIV/AIDS and ART. This approach recognises that quality NCD service delivery involves the whole district health team; and is an integrated process across the PHC level facilities and the district hospital. Countries will need to adopt and adapt the global guidelines according to the local context.

The target audience for the simple standard implementation guideline is front-line programme managers, clinicians and health providers in district health teams who are planning and delivering the NCD control interventions. An integrated document best serves the needs of clients and patients who may have linked NCDs and overlapping clinical problems; and is best suited for health workers in first- and second-level settings as it facilitates their work to deliver these linked interventions across a district, at community clinics and PHC centres and district hospitals.

As experience is gained with the roll-out of a simple set of disease packages, the guideline document can be expanded and updated with technical developments and therapeutic advances. Several can be anticipated: broader POC screening with simple hand-held devices; further interventions like the polypill and management of high cholesterol; new strategies for screening and treatment for common mental health disorders; additional biomedical interventions to manage nicotine and alcohol dependence; developments in screening for cervical and other cancers.

New medicines for weight loss are on the horizon: the first drug in the GLP-1 class, semaglutide, is already approved in the United States and prescribed in the UK on the NHS. These drugs were developed for diabetes control and have the potential to revolutionise obesity management; they may also have a role in managing alcohol dependence. They will inevitably drop in price and be made available to the global south for inclusion in NCD care guidelines.

The WHO treatment guidelines for a public health approach to scaling up ART started as a simple short document. As HIV testing and ART scaled up, staff became more experienced; prevention was included; guidelines consolidated and grew significantly in size, scope and complexity. The proposed guidelines for a public health approach to scaling up NCD control interventions in resource-limited settings are already consolidated across several main NCDs with a broad prevention and treatment focus: they will inevitably become more complex and detailed as experience is gained with their roll-out and needs evolve. Provided this is accompanied with extra resources and staffing, this is to be welcomed. However, the focus must continue to be on the district health team and the primary axis must be on patient and personal care at the PHC level.

Integrated service delivery: primary health care linked with the district hospital

Treatment guidelines for a public health approach for scaling up NCD interventions in resource-limited settings are aimed at the district health team and based on an NCD service delivery model that integrates health centres and PHC facilities with the first-level district hospital. Screening and diagnostic testing are at the PHC level or outpatient clinic. Disease management protocols for primary and secondary prevention and treatment have referral to the hospital when blood sugar or BP is not controlled; or for cancer diagnosis when signs and symptoms mandate urgent referral. Long-term clinical management is based in the community and at the primary care level.

ART started as a physician-led intervention managed from specialist units in tertiary facilities. One of the first challenges was to develop a hub-and-spoke model for service delivery that effectively integrated health centres and PHC facilities with their district hospital to make ART more equitably accessible and to facilitate rapid scale-up. This will not been an issue with NCD interventions: the challenge will be to ensure that district hospital care is included along with a very strong, sometimes almost exclusive focus on PHC.

The district health team includes clinical officers, nurses, midwives, pharmacists, practitioners in allied professions and community health workers who are based at service delivery points in the community, at PHC facilities and the district hospital. They manage upward and downward referral of patients as clinical problems arise and are managed with access to a limited range of first-line and essential medicines. They have the most patient contact, follow treatment protocols in the guidelines, and deliver health promotion messages and education about healthy living and NCD risks. Quality care delivery is predicated on their regular support and supervision. Community healthcare workers can successfully implement provider-led BP interventions (He et al., 2023).

Physicians are based in hospitals and are rarely deployed to the periphery. They can prescribe from a wider set of essential second-line and third-line medicines that are carried in better stocked hospital pharmacies; they diagnose cancers and can manage interventions not available at the PHC level; and a wide variety of blood tests and investigations like radiology and ultrasound can be performed to support complex case management. Heart attacks and stroke can be managed and stroke rehabilitation commenced for long-term community delivery. Physicians and senior hospital-based clinicians also need to supervise and support workers in peripheral facilities.

The district hospital is the hub at the centre of the team, its peripheral facilities and nodes. A well-functioning hospital will have a well-stocked district pharmacy; laboratory and radiology services; rehabilitation; and special facilities for surgery and obstetrics. Special focus may need to be given to developing some of these services, which may be run down; or establishing them in the first place: the need for rehabilitation is particularly pressing (Kamenov et al., 2019). The district management team is responsible for procurement and supply chain management; and staff supervision and support. Informal providers can improve the quality of care delivered, provided they are intensively trained and supervised (Das et al., 2016).

Having a well-staffed and functioning hospital and a strong district health team is the key minimum requirement for implementing the NCD treatment guidelines. The whole team must be resourced and supported otherwise quality will suffer and the multi-tasked front-line health workers will be overwhelmed. Special consideration and resources will need to be given to mental health services for implementing the actions in the WHO comprehensive mental health action plan; current service provision is grossly inadequate (World Health Organization (WHO), 2021a).

A strong and well-resourced district health team supported to implement NCD interventions can also accommodate and cover ongoing vertical disease control programmes like HIV/AIDS, TB and malaria; and integrate their screening and clinical management with NCD services. There may well be some economy of scale with integration of service delivery particularly as regards clinical staff time. It may also be more efficient to pool funding with resources hopefully forthcoming for NCD control. This is the obverse of current practice to integrate prevention and control of NCDs into vertical HIV/AIDS and TB programmes (World Health Organization (WHO), 2023d).

Several important services can be provided outside core NCD interventions that are what people, patients and communities expect of a functioning health service; and which include most if not all of the set of 108 highest-priority disease control interventions identified by DCP3 as implementable and providing value for money (Jamison et al., 2018): essential interventions for maternal, newborn and child health (MNCH) as part of the interventions and strategies for improving reproductive, maternal, newborn and child healthcare (Lassi et al., 2014); essential surgery at first-level district hospitals surgery (Mock et al., 2015); and as part of the continuum of care, palliative care and rehabilitation services. It can also address the Neglected Tropical Diseases (NTDs) where these are locally relevant and need concerted action (World Health Organization (WHO), 2023c).

A well-functioning district health team could also have a significant role in reducing the threat that antimicrobial resistance (AMR) poses, particularly to poor and marginalised communities. Antibiotics are often used as substitutes for basic care; when formal healthcare services are missing, patients purchase antibiotics from pharmacists or lay providers. Inappropriate use of antibiotics contributes to the emergence and spread of AMR. A district health team should adhere to treatment protocols for common infections and only prescribe approved antibiotics. Providing a limited range of essential antibiotics for free in public sector pharmacies across the district is key for antimicrobial stewardship and could significantly reduce pressures on AMR (World Health Organization (WHO), 2018a).

Pandemic preparedness and resilient health systems enabling communities to face disasters need robust health systems and services; and a functioning district health team which can respond and react to the challenge. One lesson from SARS-CoV-2/COVID-19 was how unprepared most low- and middle-income countries were to respond, and how quickly health services were overwhelmed.

Raising the resources: looking towards universal healthcare and coverage

Implementing treatment guidelines for a public health approach for scaling up NCD interventions in resource-limited settings is dependent on a district health team that is properly resourced and supported to provide quality services. Strengthened health systems are the key for equitable access to all in need, and for quality service delivery; but they are costly to set up and maintain. Without a significant upturn in funding, it is difficult to see any way to achieve SDG target 3.4 to reduce premature NCD mortality by one-third by 2030; or target 3.8 to achieve universal health coverage (UHC) by 2030.

At present, much domestic funding for health in low- and middle-income countries is provided by individual and household out-of-pocket payments which can be catastrophic particularly for chronic diseases with significant morbidity; these constitute 50% of healthcare financing in low-income countries. Health is a basic human right: it is generally accepted that the poorest people require complete subsidisation for healthcare costs from general taxes (Mills, 2014). One obvious fiscal approach is to tax unhealthy habits like smoking, excess alcohol and sugary carbonated drinks. Despite the clear health benefits, significant industry resistance has often limited the revenue that is raised through taxation. When fiscal measures are implemented, it is critical that revenue does not disappear into general services but is hypothecated to health.

Governments can also decide to raise national health budgets significantly as they aim to raise taxes on unhealthy products as both need bold political commitments to health for all as a universal human right and to PHC and UHC. They may be encouraged to increase health spend if they can refer to successful programmes and have confidence there will be a significant political and economic return: HIV/AIDS is one good example of what can be achieved.

There is an important opportunity for citizens, voters and networks of PLWNCD to exert pressure on government and create demand for accessible, effective quality NCD services. Governments can be reminded that they have made significant commitments at various UN HLMs to delivering on the NCD agenda. Patient and consumer groups can articulate community needs for stronger health systems and more accessible health services to deliver health for all and reach the poorest first, as part of the 2030 agenda for sustainable development, ratified by all UN member states. There may be an opportunity post-COVID-19 for additional revenue for health as countries build back better, plan for more resilient health systems and develop pandemic preparedness.

Development assistance for health, from bilateral and multilateral sources makes up around half of the health budgets in low-income countries. If health systems are to be strengthened to deliver quality pro-poor services and aligned with the lofty SDG aims to leaving no one behind and to reach the furthest behind first; and be better capacitated to be more resilient to disasters and pandemics, then there needs to be a significant upturn in resources for health in general and those earmarked for NCDs. High-income countries have also made significant commitments to the NCD agenda at various UN HLMs; global health practitioners and international NCD alliances must remind governments of this.

One smart way to leverage more resources could be to ask donors to match increases in domestic health budgets, and somehow link this to an extended horizon for these investments beyond the usual five-year funding cycle. It may also be time to link this to general health systems strengthening rather that any particular vertical disease control programme. Investing in strong health systems and services ensures better health outcomes across the board; a narrow investment in one programme can, as with HIV/AIDS result is outstanding outcomes, but they are restricted to one disease.

In all health systems, decision-makers must determine how to allocate limited budgets to maximise outcomes for the populations they serve. Historically there have been two approaches for resource allocation: vertical, where funding targets specific interventions and disease control programmes; and horizontal, which focusses on funding interventions like PHC or MNCH services to strengthen the health system (Frenk, 2010).

Whilst the need for health systems strengthening has been strongly made by many global health academics and some global health initiatives like GAVI, vertical approaches have dominated over the last two decades. This has been led by the exceptional global response to HIV/AIDS specifically to close the AIDS treatment gap; latterly joined by TB and malaria and strongly reflected in the MDG 2015 health targets. To some extent the SGDs perpetuate this with a further vertical focus on NCDs.

New funding mechanisms have been set up: the multilateral Global Fund to fight AIDS, TB and malaria; and the bilateral US President's Emergency Fund for AIDS Relief (PEPFAR). Billions have been invested in vertical programmes, with dramatic success, but at some cost. NCD advocates have lamented the over-concentration of resources to the "fashionable" diseases while calling for more resources for the neglected NCD epidemic (Geneau et al., 2010).

Over-concentrated resource allocation does not match the global burden of disease: well-financed vertical programmes divert skilled health professionals, in short supply in most low-income countries, away from PHC services. However, the NCD action group was clear that a new funding mechanism for NCDs is not required; instead better use of existing resources and innovative new sources of funding is mandated (Beaglehole et al., 2011).

Despite vocally highlighting the NCD crisis, extensive discussion in UN HLMs over the years and the wide promotion of cost-effective best buys, very little progress has been made; there has been no success in establishing any global vertical NCD programme that can deliver anything towards the SDG goals. Perhaps now is the time to agree that a new approach to resource mobilisation is needed by pivoting from vertical approaches to disease control towards the horizontal and to call for general investment in health system strengthening.

To support this, the Global Fund could think of rebranding itself as a Fund for Health and visibly move to a broader agenda for health and development from a rather restricted approach focussing on AIDS, TB and malaria. PEPFAR could also broaden out from an exclusive focus on HIV/AIDS and incorporate health system strengthening. These innovations will be deeply unpopular with some international NGOs and multilateral agencies like UNAIDS focussed on single issues, even as we anticipate ending AIDS by 2030. Community and civil society organisations who have been vocal champions for ART and who represent vulnerable key populations and marginalised groups may be particularly concerned that hard won successes will be reversed.

Reassurance will be needed that any such change would not result in reduced funding for disease control programmes or compromise service delivery. Instead, raising additional resources for health and channelling funds into integrated and strengthened health systems will facilitate quality service improvement and better patient-focussed and person-centred care outcomes. Community will appreciate a broader response to additional disease control priorities that are currently without a narrow vertical NCD, HIV, TB and malaria approach; and which better reflect the current and evolving burden of disability and disease.

Better integration is the next step: but it is insufficient and ultimately will be inefficient as vertical programmes tend to duplicate services and generate extra costs. By covering care needs more universally than vertical programmes can, strengthened health systems are more efficient and capable of delivering quality services that impact morbidity and mortality regardless of cause. They are also the route towards UHC.

Clearly making progress on the UHC agenda cannot happen without successful disease control programmes reducing morbidity and mortality and financial hardship; and significant progress being made with providing interventions for NCD prevention and care. But vertical disease programmes need to realise that for their long-term success and sustainability they increasingly will require more wide-ranging interventions in sectors outside of healthcare which address non-medical social and environmental determinants of health, which have long-term greater potential to improve overall health outcomes (Bloom et al., 2018).

There is a powerful justification for funding health services strengthening above and beyond the verticalised care approaches currently in place for AIDS, TB and malaria, and strongly advocated for the NCDs. This is not a threat to successful control programmes and should be the mechanism to address more effectively the NCD crisis. Instead this is the route towards delivering on UHC and broadening into social and environmental health determinants that increasingly impact health and disease.

Section 3

Delivering universal health coverage in the global south

10 Health and the universal health coverage agenda

The centrality of health in human development

Good health is essential to human welfare and to sustained social and economic development. Improvements in health can be seen as an end in themselves and crucial to overall well-being and the related concepts of capabilities and opportunities. Health can affect overall well-being directly and indirectly, for example, through income and wealth. Health can also be seen as of great importance due to its impact on people's range of opportunities – such as their ability to work or pursue an education (Helliwell & Putnam, 2004). Healthy children are better able to learn, and a healthy population facilitates economic growth (Alsan et al., 2007). Initiatives to improve the health status of people are thus not only the right thing to do, but also pragmatic approaches to human development (Marmot et al., 2008). On the other hand, poor population health contributes to social and economic instability and undermines development efforts (The Word Bank, 1993).

However, for millions of people, the right to the enjoyment of the highest attainable standard of physical and mental health, including access to medicines, remains a distant goal, especially for children and those living in poverty; hence, the likelihood of achieving this goal is becoming increasingly remote (World Health Organisation (WHO), 2013). In addition, millions of people are driven below the poverty line each year because of catastrophic out-of-pocket (OOP) payments for healthcare (Van Doorslaer et al., 2005). Excessive OOP payments also discourage the impoverished from seeking or continuing care (Falkingham, 2004).

The right to health is recognised as a fundamental human right in the World Health Organisation (WHO) Constitution. Every human being has the right to the enjoyment of the highest attainable standard of physical and mental health, without distinction and the right of everyone to a standard of living adequate for the health and well-being of oneself, including food, clothing, housing and medical care and necessary social services, and the right to security in the event of shocks or lack of livelihood in circumstances beyond one's control (World

DOI: 10.4324/9781003505693-14

Health Organization (WHO), 1946). Most nations have signed many accords, establishing that provision of health is a fundamental human right since the mid-20th century. It has been argued that countries should set specific targets and strengthen their health systems towards universal health coverage (UHC), which means that all people – no matter who they are or where they live – can receive quality health services, when and where they are needed, without incurring financial hardship (Frenk, 2009).

UHC improves population health, which in turn, contributes to development directly (Maeda et al., 2014). UHC, through a primary healthcare (PHC) approach that deals with health services in a comprehensive way, including the promotion, prevention and control of diseases, can be useful in lessening the burden of non-communicable diseases (Kieny et al., 2017). This, in turn, can also assist in lowering healthcare expenditures, which can severely limit well-being and opportunities (Donaldson et al., 2011). Affordable access across the entire continuum of care facilitates the use of preventive services, which are often more cost-effective than the corresponding curative services (Woolf, 2009).

It has become evident that sustainable development is only possible when "no one is left behind" (Ranabhat et al., 2021), where all people obtain the health services they need without risking financial hardship from unaffordable OOP payments (World Health Organization (WHO), 2010). UHC is the best way to fulfil the promise of "leaving no one behind" in the 2030 Agenda for Sustainable Development (World Health Organization (WHO), 2018c). Many institutions, including WHO, have advocated for UHC on the basis that it not only leads to better health and to financial protection but also that it is valuable for its own sake (Kutzin, 2013). The evidence suggests that UHC generally leads to better access to necessary care and improved population health, particularly for poor people (Moreno-Serra & Smith, 2012). The role of UHC in improving health, reducing poverty and driving development, and its link with a more just and equitable world are now firmly implanted (Frenk & De Ferranti, 2012). Achieving UHC is not an easy proposition; nevertheless, countries can create the conditions in which UHC is achieved and the right to health is ensured for everyone with concrete and coordinated actions at international and national levels.

In the context of weak health systems in low- and middle-income countries, approaches for delivering healthcare towards UHC has shifted over time. During the basic health services approach in the 1950s and 1960s as well as the PHC movement in the 1970s, the major foci were availability, accessibility and appropriateness (King, 1966; Rifkin, 2018; World Health Organization (WHO), 1978b). More recently, new global health initiatives have shifted the agenda of UHC to obligations that need commitments at international and national levels. It is prudent to accelerate efforts aimed at ensuring UHC for all, linking the goal with all stakeholders, and country health aspirations related to health, human rights and poverty. This effort will need working on many fronts, starting with the political will of governments and civil societies. Under the Universal Declaration of Human Rights, countries are obliged to follow core obligations including ensuring access to health facilities, goods and services to everyone. According to Article 12 of the International Covenant on Economic, Social, and Cultural Rights, adoption of a national public health strategy and plan of action is a core obligation of countries (United Nations General Assembly, 1948).

Box 10.1 Universal health coverage and universal healthcare

The term universal health coverage has most often been applied to low- and middle-income countries while the term universal healthcare has most frequently been used in describing policies for care in high-income countries. While the basic definition of UHC is conceptually straightforward and applied universally throughout the world, countries should have context-specific approaches to UHC implementation as well as a potential range of relevant metrics due to variations in countries' epidemiology, health systems and financing. Any country can take steps to progressively realize UHC, using a context-specific approach.

Improving access to health services (where services are physically accessible, financially affordable and acceptable to patients) is one such step towards UHC. Access is a general concept that summarizes a set of more specific dimensions describing the fit between the client and the health system. The specific dimensions are availability, accessibility, accommodation, affordability and acceptability. On the other hand, coverage is considered as a concept expressing the extent of interaction between the service and the people for whom it is intended. Health systems can primarily improve the health of individuals and populations by delivering accessible and high-quality interventions, also called effective coverage, to those who may benefit from them.

History of universal healthcare and coverage

UHC has been a dream for many countries since the end of the Second World War (WWII), but it became a reality only after the Alma-Ata Declaration in 1978, when the WHO called for "health for all" by the year 2000 (World Health Organization (WHO), 1979). Following WWII, universal healthcare systems began to be set up around the world. On 5 July 1948, the United Kingdom launched its universal National Health Service and founded the National Health Service (NHS), providing free care at the point of delivery to all people (Bump, 2015; Webster, 2002). The NHS is supported by taxes and continues to offer healthcare to the British people. It served as a model for many countries to emulate, and it is today regarded as one of the world's top healthcare systems (Takaku et al., 2014; Webster, 2002).

Mexico established a universal healthcare system, known as the Instituto Mexicano del Seguro Social (IMSS), in the 1960s. The IMSS provides healthcare services to employees and their families in the formal sector, while the Seguro Popular provides health insurance to individuals in the informal sector. Despite these initiatives, poor Mexicans and indigenous populations continue to confront major impediments to healthcare access. Mexico's *Seguro Popular* shows the importance of phasing in coverage innovations, beginning with the most vulnerable populations in society. Under the 2003 scheme, the most dramatic efforts targeted unemployed Mexican people and those working in the informal economy or farming (González Anaya & García Cuéllar, 2015).

In 1961, Japan implemented universal healthcare, providing a basic healthcare package to all citizens and legal residents. The Japanese system is mandatory and tax-funded, with the government determining the rates of healthcare services, which helps to keep expenses under control. It has succeeded in obtaining UHC, with about 100% of the population insured (Ikegami, 2014).

Universal health insurance was implemented in Australia in 1975 with the *Medibank*, which led to universal coverage under the current Medicare system from 1984 (Boxall, 2010). From the 1970s to the 2000s, Western European countries began introducing universal coverage, most of them building upon previous health insurance programs to cover the whole population (Bärnighausen & Sauerborn, 2002).

China began its own universal healthcare system in 1984, which has grown tremendously over the years (Yu, 2015). The strategy in the country is based on a social health insurance system that serves both urban and rural populations. However, the government still faces substantial hurdles in ensuring that all residents have equal access to high-quality healthcare services (Tan et al., 2019).

Beyond the 1990s, many countries in Latin America, the Caribbean, Africa and the Asia-Pacific region, including developing countries, took steps to bring their populations under universal health coverage, including China (Yu, 2015) and Brazil (Dimas, 2022; Muzaka, 2017). Ghana was the first nation in Africa to implement universal healthcare in 2003 when the National Health Insurance Scheme (NHIS) was put into place. All Ghanaians are intended to have access to cheap healthcare services through the NHIS, a tax-funded insurance programme (Agyepong et al., 2016).

A review on UHC concludes that reaching UHC it is not an unattainable goal reserved for high-income countries; it is achievable in middle- and upper middle-income countries. Successes and failures are seen both in the case of countries that pursue a contributory health insurance path to UHC and those that pursue a core government funding path. *De jure* constitutional guarantees and national health legislation are often necessary but do not guarantee success

without accompanying institutional measures (political and economic) and supply (service provision) and consumer/patient behaviour (demand constraints)
(Preker et al., 2021). Every country is different and needs to find its own path
towards UHC; it should learn from the achievements and failures of others.
History suggests that ensuring universal coverage takes some time; in the UK,
nearly five decades of hard work and political debate were needed. South Korea
did it faster, but still needed about two decades to attain universal coverage.
There is no timetable attached to the WHO 2005 resolution for universal health
coverage (Yates, 2009).

Universal health coverage at the World Health Organization and the United Nations

Since the mid-20th century, most nations have signed many accords, establishing that provision of health is a fundamental human right (Cerda, 1990; Craven,
1995; Union, 1997). Health for all has been not only an aspirational target but
also an essential framework for the United Nations system. The constitution of
the WHO asserts that a right to health is "one of the fundamental rights of every
human being without distinction of race, religion, political belief, economic or
social condition" (World Health Organization (WHO), 1946). This message has
been repeatedly reinforced perhaps most prominently since the 1978 Declaration
of Alma-Ata. UHC was firmly endorsed, as a central goal, by the World Health
Assembly in 2005 (World Health Organization (WHO), 2005b) and further supported in the World Health Report 2010 (World Health Organization (WHO),
2010).

In 2005, the member states of WHO stated that health systems must be further
developed in order to guarantee access to necessary services while providing
protection against financial risk (World Health Organization (WHO), 2005b).
In 2005, Member States of WHO committed to UHC so that all, irrespective
of background, have access to the health services they need without suffering
financial hardship (World Health Organization (WHO), 2005b). The World
Health Report 2010, entitled "Health systems financing: the path to universal
coverage" reaffirm the importance of UHC, followed up by providing practical
guidance for how countries can reform their health financing systems to pursue
UHC (World Health Organization (WHO), 2010).

In 2011, the World Health Assembly responded by calling on WHO to develop
a plan of action for providing such support and advice. One of the action plan's
12 points is action on equity, a key issue that cuts across most other components
of a health system. Specifically, the WHO Consultative Group on Equity and
Universal Health Coverage was set up to develop guidance on how countries
best can address the central issues of fairness and equity that arise on the path to
UHC. Since 2011, the pressing need to make progress towards UHC has been
repeatedly affirmed (World Health Organisation (WHO), 2011).

On 12 December 2012, the United Nations General Assembly endorsed a resolution on Global Health and Foreign Policy urging countries to accelerate progress towards UHC, as an essential priority for international development. Member states also recognized that the importance of universal coverage in national health systems, especially through PHC and social protection mechanisms, to provide access to health services for all, in particular for the poorest segments of the population (United Nations General Assembly, 2012). Moreover, in late 2012, the United Nations General Assembly adopted a resolution emphasizing the responsibility of governments to "urgently and significantly scale up efforts to accelerate the transition towards universal access to affordable and quality health-care services." They emphasised the need to promote physical and mental health and well-being and extend life expectancy for all through UHC without leaving anyone behind (United Nations General Assembly, 2012).

Later, WHO published the World Health Report 2013, Research for Universal Health Coverage, which again emphasized the need to make progress towards UHC and described several means to that end. Advancing UHC has been identified as a leadership priority for WHO in the 12th general programme of work during the 2014–2019 period. UHC is also a central theme in the ongoing deliberation over the post-2015 development agenda. Many countries have intensified their efforts in progressing towards UHC. The results have been encouraging and supported the Director-General's assertion that UHC is "the single most powerful concept that public health has to offer."

On 25 September 2015, the resolution on Transforming Our World: the 2030 Agenda for Sustainable Development adopted the target of UHC by 2030, including financial risk protection, access to quality essential healthcare services and access to safe, effective, quality and affordable essential medicines and vaccines for all (United Nations General Assembly, 2015). The 2030 agenda for sustainable development includes health as a central component of development; the third sustainable development goal (SDG-3) aims to ensure healthy lives and promote well-being for all at all ages. UHC has been set as an umbrella target for health in the post-2015 development agenda. SDG-3 has a specific target on UHC (target 3.8). Target 3.8.1 captures the service coverage dimension of UHC (that everyone – irrespective of their living standards – should receive the health services they need). Target 3.8.2 captures the population exposed to financial hardship due to OOP payments made when using health services through the incidence of catastrophic health spending. In addition, the incidence of impoverishing OOP spending is used to identify the extent to which payments at point of use contribute to poverty.

On 12 December 2017, the UN passed a third resolution on Global Health and Foreign Policy: addressing the health of the most vulnerable for an inclusive society, which called on Member States to promote and strengthen their dialogue with other stakeholders, including civil society, academia and the private sector, in order to maximize their engagement in and contribution to the implementation of health goals and targets through an intersectoral and multi-stakeholder approach. Since 2017, 12 December has been proclaimed by the UN as International Universal Health Coverage Day, which aims to raise awareness of the need for strong and resilient health systems and UHC with multi-stakeholder partners. Each year on 12 December, UHC advocates raise their voices to share the stories of the millions of people still waiting for health, champion what has been achieved so far, call on leaders to make bigger and smarter investments in health, and encourage diverse groups to make commitments to help move the world closer to UHC by 2030.

In 2018, WHO released its 13th general programme of work to achieve SDG-3. The program of work aims to address three interlinked goals: achieving UHC – 1 billion more people benefitting from UHC; addressing health emergencies – 1 billion more people better protected from public health emergencies; and promoting healthier populations – 1 billion more people enjoying better health and well-being (World Health Organization (WHO), 2018e).

UHC is about ensuring that all people have access to quality health services according to need while also ensuring that the use of these services does not expose the user to financial hardship (World Health Organization (WHO), 2015, 2017b). This is possible by increasing the proportion of the population that accesses quality services and decreasing the proportion of the population that spends a large amount of household income on health (Kieny & Evans, 2013). Currently, there is consensus about "why and what" for UHC. There is, however, considerable debate about "how" to achieve UHC what strategies are feasible and effective towards UHC (Horton & Das, 2015).

In September 2019, at the United Nations High-Level Meeting (UN HLM) "Universal Health Coverage: Moving Together to Build a Healthier World," world leaders endorsed the most ambitious and comprehensive political declaration on health in history. In doing so, they committed to ensuring that by 2030 everyone in their country will receive all the quality health services they need without suffering financial hardship. They reaffirmed that health is a precondition for and an outcome and indicator of the social, economic and environmental dimensions of sustainable development and the implementation of the 2030 Agenda for Sustainable Development, and strongly recommit to achieve UHC by 2030.

In September 2023, the 78th United Nations General Assembly held three UN HLM on health. The 2023 UN HLM on UHC provides countries and stakeholders an opportunity to reinvigorate progress towards delivering health for all. To ensure implementation and accountability, an action-oriented outcome that builds on the 2019 Political Declaration focusing on creating resilient and equitable health systems, with PHC as a foundation. The theme for the UN HLM on UHC is: UHC: expanding our ambition for health and well-being in a post-COVID world. It recognizes the consequence of the adverse impact of climate change, natural disasters, extreme weather events as well as the need to improve other environmental determinants of health, such as clean air, safe drinking water, sanitation, safe, sufficient and nutritious food and shelter. Hence, they underscore the need to foster health in climate change adaptation efforts, underlining that resilient and people-centred health systems are necessary to protect the health of all people, in particular those who are vulnerable or in vulnerable situations.

Dimensions and monitoring indicators of universal health coverage

Figure 10.1 depicts the three dimensions of UHC. Every country must make progress in at least three dimensions to achieve UHC. These three dimensions closely correspond to those often emphasized in the context of financing. The dimensions are related to (a) the proportion of the population to be covered, (b) the range of services to be made available and (c) the proportion of the total costs to be met (Watkins et al., 2018). In each dimension, countries moving forward will face at least one critical choice regarding fairness and equity. When expanding priority services, countries must decide which services to expand first. It is generally helpful to begin with cost-effectiveness estimates and then incorporate concern for the less fortunate as well as other relevant variables (Cookson et al., 2017). Services can then be divided into three categories: high-priority, medium-priority and low-priority (Norheim, 2015). When including more people, countries must decide whom to include first. To incorporate more people equally, countries should first expand coverage for low-income groups and other

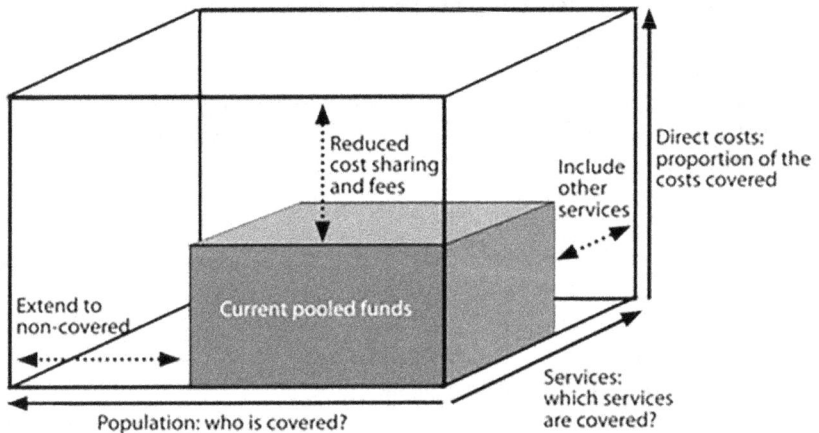

Figure 10.1 The three dimensions of universal health coverage

groups that are disadvantaged in terms of service coverage, health, or both. This is particularly critical for high-priority services (Norheim, 2015).

When reducing OOP payments, countries must decide how to shift from OOP payment towards prepayment (Boerma et al., 2014). Access to services should be based on need and not ability to pay. To improve access and financial risk protection, countries should shift from OOP payment towards mandatory prepayment with pooling of funds (Tandon & Reddy, 2021). OOP payments should first be reduced for high-priority services and for disadvantaged groups. Mandatory prepayments should generally increase with ability to pay and be progressive (Norheim, 2015).

The UHC monitoring framework developed by WHO and the World Bank (Boerma et al., 2014) proposes that measurement of coverage with financial risk protection be conducted simultaneously with measurement of coverage with essential prevention and treatment services. Indicators of essential services coverage include a quality component referred to as effective coverage in addition to the proportion of the population that makes contact with the service of interest (contact coverage) (Tanahashi, 1978). Effective coverage adjusts contact coverage using a weight that reflects the quality of service being offered according to the standard guidelines. A third feature of UHC, in addition to effective coverage and financial risk protection, is universality which aims coverage for everyone (Evans et al., 2013).

The SDGs have two indicators for its 3.8 target on service coverage (SDG 3.8.1) and financial protection (SDG 3.8.2).

- Indicators of service coverage (SDG 3.8.1)

   The goal of achieving UHC includes ensuring that all individuals have access to the necessary health services to improve their well-being. The inclusive nature of UHC and its emphasis on providing health services of sufficient quality to be effective to those in need poses unique challenges for monitoring service coverage. That means, one single index cannot fully capture all of the health services described in the definition of UHC. Four principles guided the development of the UHC index construction: coverage of main health areas; inclusion of different types of services (health promotion, illness prevention, curative services, rehabilitation, palliative services); preference for effective coverage measures if available; and whether disaggregation was possible by key dimensions of inequality (Hogan et al., 2018). It is measured through a service coverage index (SCI), which takes into account various indicators, such as reproductive, maternal and child health, infectious diseases, noncommunicable diseases and access to services. However, monitoring service coverage for UHC is challenging due to its inclusive nature and focus on providing high-quality services throughout one's life. As a result, the current SCI uses a selection of indicators to represent the overall coverage of essential health services across a country's entire population. It is calculated

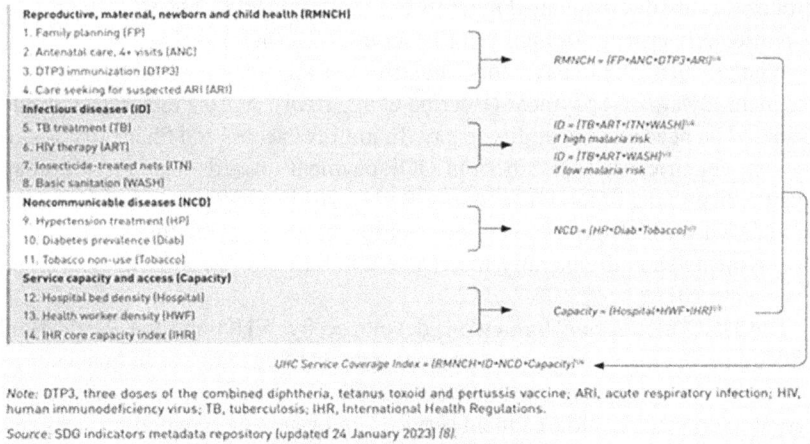

Figure 10.2 Calculation of universal health coverage service coverage index (SDG 3.8.1)

as the geometric mean of 14 indicators and sub-grouped in four categories (Figure 10.2).

• Indicators of financial protection (SDG 3.8.2)

The goal of UHC pertains not only to access to health services but is also centrally concerned with affordability and financial protection beyond their role as barriers to access. Three measures are particularly relevant indicators of financial risk linked to OOP payments: proportion of OOP payments, percentage of the total population that faces catastrophic health expenditure due to OOP payments, and percentage of the total population impoverished due to OOP payments.

Box 10.2 Indicators of financial protection

Proportion of OOP payments: This is defined as the proportion of OOP payments relative to the total health expenditure. The proportion of OOP payments is primarily linked to financial risk protection by a known high correlation between that proportion and catastrophic health expenditure and impoverishment. Evidence suggests that OOP payments typically have to represent less than 15 to 20 percent of total health expenditure before the incidence of catastrophic health expenditures and impoverishment falls to negligible levels.

Percentage of the total population that faces catastrophic health expenditure due to OOP payments: Health expenditures are typically considered catastrophic for a household if they exceed a certain threshold, for example, 40 percent of non-food household expenditures in a year.

Percentage of the total population impoverished due to OOP payments: Impoverishing OOP payment is defined as the proportion of the population, over a year, that is pushed below the poverty line due to OOP payments.

Universal health coverage and health security

UHC and health security are concepts that are intertwined and mutually beneficial (Assefa, Hill, Gilks, Damme, et al., 2020; Kutzin & Sparkes, 2016). UHC aspires to give all persons, regardless of capacity to pay, with access to high-quality healthcare services, whereas health security focuses on ensuring that communities are prepared for and protected against shocks, including infectious disease outbreaks, bioterrorism and other health emergencies. These strategic priorities require implementation that is jointly reinforcing. However, there is insufficient reconciliation and tension between global health security (GHS) and UHC towards a healthier and safer world (Ooms et al., 2017, 2018). In addition, there are disagreements within the broader GHS community on security from what kind of health threat, security for whom and how (Rushton, 2011).

The COVID-19 pandemic has underlined the significance of UHC and health security in maintaining the health and well-being of individuals and communities worldwide (World Health Organization (WHO), 2021a). Countries with strong health systems, especially those that have invested in UHC and health security, have been better positioned to prevent and mitigate the virus's spread, whereas others with weaker health systems have struggled to deal with the pandemic (World Health Organization (WHO), 2021a).

UHC and health security have various synergies (Agyepong et al., 2023; Verrecchia et al., 2019). UHC can improve disease identification and response by increasing access to healthcare services. Individuals are more likely to seek medical assistance for symptoms and illnesses if they have access to healthcare services, lowering the chance of untreated infections spreading to others. Similarly, health security activities, such as immunisation programmes can be utilised to target underserved groups, enhancing UHC and lowering the risk of disease outbreaks (Sarker et al., 2022).

UHC and health security can also be strengthened by strengthening healthcare personnel training and capacity. Healthcare systems can increase their ability to respond to infectious illnesses and other health emergencies by investing in healthcare worker training and ensuring that they have the required skills and resources. In addition to these synergies, UHC and health security programmes can share resources and infrastructure. For example, health security efforts, such as emergency stockpiles of medical supplies and equipment can be utilised to support UHC programmes during non-emergency times, ensuring that healthcare services remain available and of good quality.

Conversely, UHC initiatives can aid in health security efforts by boosting access to diagnostics and testing (Lal et al., 2022). UHC can improve disease surveillance and response by boosting access to these resources, as well as aid in the early discovery of outbreaks. UHC and health security measures can also work jointly to address health equity. UHC can help to eliminate health inequities, especially those that put certain communities at greater risk of infectious disease, by enhancing access to healthcare services. Similarly, health security programmes can address underlying social determinants of health, such as poverty and poor housing, which can contribute to the spread of infectious disease (Assefa, Hill, Gilks, Damme, et al., 2020).

11 Strategies for achieving universal health coverage

Gaining and sustaining political commitment

A redistributive policy such as universal health coverage (UHC) is unlikely to happen without domestic political support. Universal health coverage is intensely political and depends on the features of a country's governance. Politics, including governance and decision-making, can support or hinder UHC (Greer & Méndez, 2015). The adoption of and commitment to UHC is a political process driven by a variety of social forces to create public programmes (Savedoff et al., 2012).

The United Nations High-Level Meeting on Universal Health Coverage: Moving Together to Build a Healthier World (2019) provided important reaffirmation of health as a precondition for sustainable development and equity. The SDG declaration provides a global political commitment and an enabling environment for putting in place necessary legislations, revisions of national health policies and reforming health financing systems to align to the country's vision towards UHC (Odoch et al., 2021).

There is growing recognition that achieving UHC is a political challenge. Interests, ideas and institutions shape UHC; that means a political understanding of UHC is needed to achieve health for all (Ho et al., 2022). It is also important to analyse the politics of health reform for UHC according to the policy cycle (agenda setting, design, adoption and implementation) and variables that affect reform (interests, institutions, ideas and ideology) (Fox & Reich, 2015). Windows of political opportunity should be utilised to ensure that UHC is set into the political agenda, and hold political parties and government accountable. This will be facilitated if UHC is considered as citizen's rights and entitlements to health through full subsidies for the poor and vulnerable populations (Berhan et al., 2022; Tangcharoensathien et al., 2021).

A lesson from Ghana indicates that advocacy is crucial to get health financing on the political agenda (Novignon et al., 2021). UHC was a political manifesto of the 2001 election campaign in Thailand. The government legislated to use general taxation as the sole source of financing for the universal

DOI: 10.4324/9781003505693-15

coverage scheme. Adequate funding for UHC was achieved, providing access to services and financial protection for vulnerable populations. Out-of-pocket (OOP) expenditure, medical impoverishment and catastrophic health spending among households decreased between 2000 and 2015. Domestic government health expenditure, strong political commitment and historical precedence of the tax-financed medical welfare scheme were key to achieving UHC in Thailand. This has been possible through transparency, multi-stakeholder engagement and use of evidence informed budgetary negotiations (Tangcharoensathien, Thammatach-Aree, et al., 2020).

Strengthening health systems, including core public health capacities

A recent evaluation of options for achieving UHC in Africa found that improving health systems is critical to achieving UHC. Many countries have begun to restructure and strengthen their health systems to achieve UHC (Jaca et al., 2022). There is a global consensus on the need for strong health systems towards UHC and tackling emerging diseases. Health system strengthening refers to significant and purposeful effort to improve the system's performance. Strengthening is one way to ensure that the system's performance embodies the intermediary objectives of health policies, plans and strategies – quality, equity, efficiency, accountability, resilience and sustainability (Kutzin & Sparkes, 2016).

Health system strengthening is a means to progress towards UHC. Functional health systems, which are strong and resilient, ensure access to and quality of essential health services, create demand for essential services and respond to shocks (Karamagi et al., 2021). A functioning health system is organised around the people, institutions and resources that are mandated to improve, maintain, or restore the health of a given population (Kieny et al., 2017). The evidence around the world proves that health systems are crucial for attaining UHC, including equity and quality (World Health Organization (WHO), 2017a). Provision of quality care is vital to improve utilisation of health services and maintain continuity of care (Sobel et al., 2016).

Almost all countries are experiencing epidemiologic overlaps between NCDs and infectious diseases (Misganaw, 2020; Tollman et al., 2008). This epidemiologic overlaps demand a health systems transition that integrates health services towards UHC (Shiferaw et al., 2018). Understanding of these dynamics is important to improve service delivery and achieve UHC as well as better health outcomes. These require a range of skills, including teamwork, partnerships and collaboration with community groups and across different sectors (Haregu et al., 2014; Letebo & Shiferaw, 2016).

The epidemiologic overlap demands health systems approaches that integrate health services towards UHC as well as improvements in poverty reduction, fertility and education (Assefa, Hill, Gilks, Admassu, et al., 2020). Health systems strengthening based on a knowledge of the epidemiology and health systems context requires a political will to invest more and better in primary healthcare (PHC) systems through a "whole-of-government" and a "whole-of-society" approaches towards UHC and health security (Berhan et al., 2022; Kraef & Kallestrup, 2019). As noted in Sections 1 and 2, to optimise care outputs and reduce disability, morbidity and premature mortality, PHC needs to be integrated with hospital services in the district health team.

The response to public health emergencies necessitates resilient (public) health systems capable of adequately preventing, detecting and responding. Countries require a unified national health system, including public health, to prevent or contain avoidable outbreaks and epidemics while simultaneously providing accessible and inexpensive healthcare (Erondu et al., 2018). However, the present International Health Regulations (2005) architecture, standards for public health functions, and frameworks for building health systems are fragmented (Balabanova et al., 2010), which has negatively affected the progress towards UHC and health security.

Such fragmentation is particularly common in low- and middle-income countries. Cognisant of this challenge, countries, such as Ethiopia, have applied synergistic approaches, including harmonisation and alignment of the national strategic plan with international commitments, to unite efforts for UHC, health security and health promotion (Tadesse et al., 2021). This should be expanded to include universal and comprehensive health systems that combine basic public health capabilities to prevent and control the next pandemic. This necessitates political will to invest in health systems and basic public health capacities in the pursuit of UHC and health security (Lal et al., 2021).

Preparing an essential benefits package: The goal of UHC is to ensure that everyone has access to critical health treatments without financial barriers. It is made up of two parts: offering a comprehensive range of high-quality health services tailored to individual requirements, and protecting persons from financial difficulty when paying for healthcare (Boerma et al., 2014). A central requirement of any system of UHC is that the services made available to the population are consistent with the funds available. While countries are pursuing fair and progressive realisation of UHC, it is crucial that choices, of services to be included in the UHC scheme, are made carefully.

The set of health services to be made available can be determined by burden of diseases and available prioritised interventions; however, its total size will be constrained by the available funds, which will limit number of services to be provided to citizens in a sustainable manner. Hence, rationing and setting priorities for the selection of interventions to be included in a defined essential benefits package (EBP) is critical (Verguet et al., 2021). An explicit essential health services benefits plan (EHSBP) – a set of health services and products that can be feasibly financed and provided for everyone in the country – is an essential element in creating a sustainable system for UHC (Glassman et al., 2017).

Designing and implementing a publicly funded EHSBP is a steppingstone towards UHC. The design should be impartial (aiming for universality), democratic (inclusive with public involvement and disadvantaged populations), based on national values and clearly defined criteria, data driven and evidence-based (while also respecting the difference between data, dialogue and decision), linked to robust financing mechanisms, providing effective service delivery mechanisms that can promote quality care, as well as open and transparent in all steps of the process and decisions (World Health Organization (WHO), 2021c). It is commendable that Ethiopia has recently developed its EHSBP. It is crucial that this plan is financed, implemented, monitored and evaluated to progressively realise UHC in the country (Eregata et al., 2020). There is, however, a significant gap in health financing to provide essential health services, according to the EHSBP. It is, thus, necessary to increase the total government health expenditure which could partly address the gap (Hailu et al., 2021).

Aiming for a progressive realisation of UHC: Progressive realisation, defined as the governmental obligations to immediately and progressively move towards the full realisation of UHC (Baltussen et al., 2017) is stated as the guiding principle on the path to UHC (Neelsen & O'Donnell, 2017). A fair and progressive realisation of UHC requires tough policy decisions, based on evidence and transparent processes that can facilitate decisions, to progressively realise UHC and the right to health (Pablos-Mendez et al., 2016). Countries should prioritise investments in a step-by-step strategy to achieve fair and progressive UHC.

Services should be classified according to societal principles such as cost-efficiency, meeting the needs of the most vulnerable, providing financial security, and assuring safety and efficacy. Focusing on cost-effective strategies that assist underprivileged populations in terms of both health and socio-economic status is critical. In this process, disadvantaged groups such as the poor, vulnerable and rural communities should not be overlooked (Baltussen et al., 2017).

It is critical that countries ensure coverage for high-priority care by eliminating out-of-pocket payments for high-priority services and expanding coverage for the most vulnerable people. It is critical that the financing system evolves as it transitions from OOP payment to required prepayment. This necessitates the creation of a plan with an engaged involvement of citizens and other key stakeholders (Eregata et al., 2020; Tangcharoensathien et al., 2017).

Improving health financing: Enhanced public financing provides the biggest improvement in health system functionality compared to OOP expenditure, which is negatively correlated with health system functionality (Karamagi et al., 2021). OOP expenses place a devastating financial strain on households, particularly those with chronic diseases. To offer protection from financial risks for the needy and those with chronic diseases, expanded coverage must go hand in hand with the establishment of sound prepayment and risk pooling arrangements (Tolla et al., 2017).

Achieving UHC requires health financing reforms (Fan & Savedoff, 2014; Odoch et al., 2021), which should increase the share of pooled health spending rather than OOP (Savedoff et al., 2012) by raising sufficient resources for health by leveraging more domestic resources (Kutzin, 2008). This depends on a growth in national incomes and a concurrent rise in health spending. It is also vital that the UHC system is reducing financial risks and barriers to care through reducing direct payments, risk pooling and prepayment (Kutzin, 2008, 2013).

The vision towards UHC demands an appropriate balance between extending coverage to more people, offering more services, and/or covering more of the cost of care (Kutzin, 2008). It requires not only more money for health but also more value for the money through effective strategic purchasing and addressing the main drivers of inefficiency, including those arising from fragmentation and duplication among actors, including donors, the government and other recipients (Bennett et al., 2010). A significant lesson from real-world data and country experience in the implementation of UHC plans is that public financing is critical towards UHC and in closing the gap (Wang et al., 2018a).

Bolstering innovation and research towards UHC: A functional health research system is a prerequisite for the achievement of UHC (Kirigia et al., 2015). The aspiration for UHC requires health system innovations and reforms supported by political, financial and technical investment. Accelerating these reforms and transition involves investment in research and innovation in which creativity is harnessed by the highest-quality science to deliver affordable, quality health services and better health for everyone (Franz & Ghebreyesus, 2019).

The WHO's 2013 World Health Report argues that a wide variety of well-designed research – ranging from clinical investigations to health policy and systems research – is needed towards a progressive realisation of UHC (Harries et al., 2015). It is vital that low- and middle-income countries are setting up networks of national observatory that would provide a mechanism for monitoring research and innovation, coordinating these efforts, and raising and distributing funds. Domestic financing will be crucial to realising sustainable progress in strengthening health research systems for the generation of local and contextualised solutions towards UHC (Rusakaniko et al., 2019).

Leveraging the private health sector towards UHC: The private sector (non-state providers) plays a significant role in the health system, including the provision of health services, medications and medical products, financial products, health workforce training, information technology, infrastructure and support services (Clarke et al., 2019). The private sector's role in healthcare is growing in scale and scope. It is thus not an option to ignore the private sector in national efforts towards UHC (Clarke et al., 2019). However, there is inadequate communication, coordination and referral of patients between private and public sectors. There is also insufficient monitoring, supervision and regulation of the private sector by public health authorities (Reta & Simachew, 2018). There is evidence that health professionals are not regulated well due to limited capacity. These have effects on the country's progress towards UHC (Dejene et al., 2019).

Making maximum use of existing human and other resources in non-state providers and correctly managing them is a crucial strategy for progressing towards UHC. Engaging non-state providers can also help to expand coverage of publicly funded health services in underserved geographic areas and with difficult-to-reach populations (Rao et al., 2018). Payment for performance has the potential to accelerate progress towards UHC by increasing service coverage and quality while decreasing user costs. This must, however, be balanced against the danger of lower coverage and quality of non-targeted treatments, which could jeopardise UHC (Binyaruka et al., 2015).

Countries must develop laws and legislation tailored to their specific circumstances in order to achieve UHC. They must also devise mechanisms to hold themselves accountable for any public-private partnerships formed. Countries should utilise a combination of legal and financial regulatory mechanisms when adopting policies on the involvement of the private sector in UHC. It is critical to recognise that the private sector is diverse, with many different types of actors. As a result, in order to build policies and programmes regarding the role of the private sector in achieving UHC, it is required to identify and interact with various private sector actors through dialogues (Clarke et al., 2019). The performance of the private sector is intrinsically linked to the structure and performance of the public sector; hence, it is imperative that the private sector regulatory response is integrated with that of the public health sector (Morgan et al., 2016). It should also be noted that involvement to the private sector requires capacity building for active supervision, monitoring, evaluation and stewardship of health services provided at various levels of providers (both public and private) (Etiaba et al., 2018).

Enhancing a primary health care approach

There is a general consensus that UHC can only be sustainably achieved with a stronger emphasis on PHC, which is placed at the centre of efforts to improve health and well-being (Takahashi, 2016). In the World Health Report 2000, PHC was acknowledged as a precursor of the new universalism to provide high-quality essential healthcare (Hill, 2018; World Health Organization (WHO), 2000). The essential values of PHC, including social justice, the right to better health for all, participation, and solidarity, have also endured the test of time (World Health Organization (WHO), 1978a). These values were also rearticulated in World Health Report 2008 by emphasising universal access and social protection through universal coverage; people-centred, responsive, integrated service delivery; health policy across all sectors; and inclusive, participatory, accountable leadership (World Health Organization (WHO), 2008).

PHC is a holistic approach that extends beyond the standard healthcare system and entails collaboration and cooperation across all sectors of society. It emphasises the importance of empowering individuals and communities while also recognising the critical role of primary care and key public health functions in the delivery of integrated health services. It recognises that health is influenced by a variety of elements such as social, economic and environmental situations, necessitating a comprehensive and collaborative response (Chotchoungchatchai et al., 2020; WHO, 1978). As the foundation of integrated health services, the third component is primary care and key public health functions.

Primary care: It emphasises comprehensive, ongoing and coordinated treatment that is accessible to all persons and treats a wide range of health conditions. Disease prevention, health promotion, surveillance and response to public health emergencies are all essential public health tasks. The evidence also shows that primary care is associated with a more equitable distribution of health in populations (Atun, 2004; Starfield et al., 2005). Hence, PHC creates the foundation for the achievement of UHC and the health-related SDGs. It is the interface for continuum of services, including health promotion, disease prevention, screening, testing, diagnosis, as well as treatment and care.

In the Solomon Islands Integrated service delivery packages, which defined the clinical and public health services that should be provided at different levels of the health system, have become key tools to operationalise the government's policy towards a more efficient, equitable, quality and sustainable health system to realise UHC (Whiting et al., 2016). Ethiopia has a flagship PHC program based on its community health extension program. The HEP enabled Ethiopia to achieve significant improvements in maternal and child health, communicable diseases, hygiene and sanitation, knowledge and healthcare seeking. The community has been a key player in the successful implementation of the HEP (Assefa et al., 2019).

Community empowerment: Empowered individuals and communities have the information, resources and support they need to actively participate in health decisions and take control of their own health outcomes. Empowerment entails education, awareness, and access to health services, as well as the ability to advocate for their rights and needs (De Vos et al., 2009; Erku et al., 2023a; Meleis, 1992; Morgan, 2001; Rifkin, 2009).

Addressing social determinants of health: Multisectoral policy and action is an initial component of PHC towards a universal and affordable access to healthcare which enables countries to realise UHC. Health care alone is insufficient for keeping people healthy and safe. Health-related policies and activities should be incorporated into the policies and actions of other sectors such as education, agriculture, housing and transportation. Multisectoral measures that can positively impact health include, for example, promoting healthy food choices in schools and introducing smoke-free rules in public places (R. B. Khatri et al., 2023; World Health Organization (WHO), 2018b). To accomplish UHC, ensure health and promote well-being, public health services such as surveillance, clean air, potable water, sanitation, vector control and tobacco control are required.

Furthermore, promoting and creating health and happiness necessitates action to enhance people's living, working and social environments (Heymann & Hertzman,

2006). Social determinants, including housing, employment, education and equity, are vital towards UHC and improved health status. Healthcare, public health and social determinants are essential conditions for good health (Gostin, 2021). Progresses towards UHC depends on enhancing community engagement as well as socio-economic development (multisectoral action to improve the living and working conditions), and its equitable distribution (Kraef & Kallestrup, 2019). Efforts to improve access, acceptability, utilisation and impact should address the need for more general outreach and social networks, according to the PHC approach, rather than a sole focus on facility-based health services (Kushitor et al., 2019).

Reinforcing digital health technologies for UHC

Innovative approaches such as digital health (DH) could advance the attainment of UHC. The World Health Organization recently put forth a Global Strategy on Digital Health, 2020–2025 (World Health Organization (WHO), 2021b). Primary care facilities with better digital literacy, motivated staff and adequate funding demonstrated a higher adoption of eHealth technologies, leading to improved, coordinated service delivery and higher patient satisfaction (Erku et al., 2023b).

Reaping the benefits of DH requires a number of actions. First, coordinated approaches, involving strong governance, regulatory mechanisms, development of appropriate policies, strategies, guidelines and toolkits, are required. Second, development and implementation of legal frameworks that will guide DH data ownership, availability, security and consent for use are also required. Third, use of context-specific DH in the presence of strong health systems, resilient communities and the social determinants of health are also critical to realise the potential of DH. Fourth, evaluation of the outcomes, impact and cost-effectiveness, together with sustainable funding models for DH are also required to inform decisions to prioritise DH (Blaya et al., 2010; Tomlinson et al., 2013). Fifth, it is imperative to train a critical mass of human resource for managing and maintaining the DH architecture and infrastructure (Tran Ngoc et al., 2018). Sixth, the end-users of DH need to be engaged in DH initiatives. Seventh, it is important to learn and adopt lessons from the successful deployment of DH technologies in other similar settings (Drury et al., 2018).

However, it is crucial to recognise that DH is not a panacea. Other conditions, such as overall leadership understanding and commitment, are critical in promoting the implementation of long-term digital solutions. Strong health systems and resilient communities are also required, as well as access to the social, economic and environmental determinants of health. Furthermore, it is critical that DH programmes should not redirect scarce human and financial resources away from health services. Deploying DH necessitates both intrinsic and extrinsic contributions from health systems, as well as high-level political commitment, national ownership and coordination, planning, implementation, monitoring and evaluation capabilities.

12 Progress and challenges for universal health coverage

Universal health services coverage: global progress and challenges

This summary of progress and challenges towards universal health coverage (UHC) is based on the 2023 UHC global monitoring report (World Health Organization (WHO), 2023). The report indicates that there was global progress towards universal health services coverage (UHSC) until the emergence of the COVID-19 pandemic. The global UHC score increased from 45 to 68, with the most significant improvements in the WHO African Region between 2000 and 2021. The scores varied across Member States, ranging from 28 to 91 in 2021. The highest regional scores were in the European Region (81) and the Region of the Americas (80), followed by the Western Pacific (79), Southeast Asia (62), Eastern Mediterranean (57) and African (44) Regions. Country-level index scores saw a range of less than 1 to 39 points of improvement, with 85 countries showing a 20–29 points increase from the 2000 baseline. The most significant improvements have been seen in the coverage of infectious diseases. The progress in UHC is largely due to the expansion of HIV antiretroviral treatment (ART) coverage, which accounted for most of the overall index score improvement. This was possible through the public health approach to ART delivery in low- and middle-income countries (World Health Organization (WHO), 2023) (Figure 12.1).

Low- and middle-income countries have made significant improvements in UHSC. While there have been gains in service coverage globally, progress has slowed down in recent years. Most countries have either worsened or shown no significant change in service coverage since the launch of the sustainable development goals in 2015. In 2021, there was still significant variation in UHSC index scores across countries, with higher income countries more likely to have higher scores. While more countries had higher service coverage levels in 2021 compared to 2000, the pace of improvement has slowed. The trend towards global equality in service coverage reversed after 2015, except in the WHO African and Southeast Asian Regions where country-level scores continued to converge (World Health Organization (WHO), 2023).

DOI: 10.4324/9781003505693-16

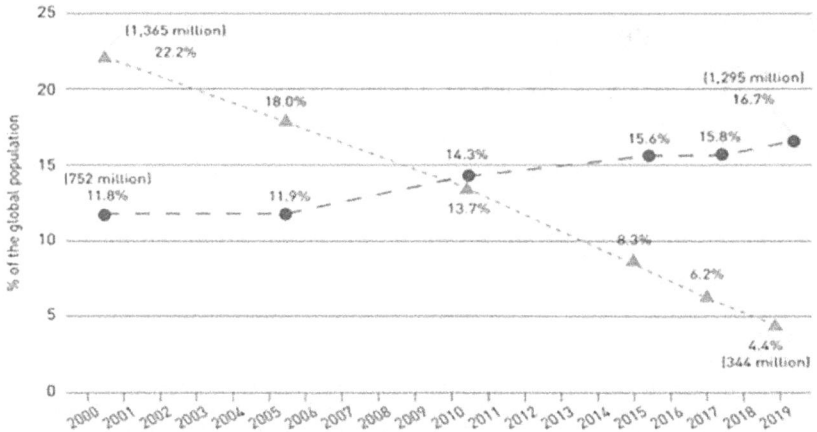

Figure 12.1 SDG 3.8.1 UHC service coverage, 2000–2021

Although the proportion of the population without essential health services has decreased since 2000, the expansion of service coverage has slowed down since 2015, and in most countries, there have been no significant improvements since 2019. A significant majority (108 out of 194 countries) have reported either a decline or no substantial change in service coverage since 2015. Around four and a half billion people worldwide are not fully covered by essential health services. Urgent political action is needed to address this situation and accelerate the expansion of all essential health services, particularly for non-communicable diseases (World Health Organization (WHO), 2023). Half of the world's population is not covered by essential health services, and billions of people experience financial hardship due to health expenses. The proportion of the population without access to essential health services decreased by 15% between 2000 and 2021, but progress has been minimal since 2015. This means that in 2021, around 4.5 billion people still did not have access to these services (World Health Organization (WHO), 2023).

Inequities in health service coverage continue to be a significant challenge for UHC. Since 2000, there has been a convergence in country-level estimates of UHSC, with lower scoring countries making progress. Between-country inequality decreased globally and in all regions from 2000 to 2015, but after 2015, inequity increased in regions other than Southeast Asia and Africa. There were also increased inequalities in TB treatment and DTP3 immunisations between countries. Inequalities in service coverage also exist within countries, highlighting the need to monitor and address disparities. However, there is limited availability of disaggregated data by age, sex and economic status (World Health Organization (WHO), 2023).

Even when there is progress at the national level, there are inequities within countries. For example, wealthier, more educated individuals living in urban areas tend to have better access to reproductive, maternal, child and adolescent health services, especially in low-income countries. Financial hardship is more common among those in poorer households and households with older family members, leading to OOP payments for healthcare. There are significant dispari-ties in reproductive, maternal, newborn and child service coverage, favouring richer households, those with more education and urban areas. The potential impact of eliminating economic-related inequalities in service coverage is sub-stantial. More data are needed on gender inequalities, socio-economic disadvan-tages and specific issues faced by indigenous peoples, refugees and migrants (World Health Organization (WHO), 2023). Within-country inequalities in UHSC should be monitored based on household economic status, education and place of residence (World Health Organization (WHO), 2023).

Financial risk protection: global progress and challenges

Out-of-pocket spending: Although most countries have shown improvements in service coverage since 2000, the situation regarding catastrophic out-of-pocket (OOP) health spending has remained unchanged or worsened for the major-ity (World Health Organization (WHO), 2023). Only a small number of coun-tries have successfully managed to enhance service coverage while reducing catastrophic OOP health spending (World Health Organization (WHO), 2023). Out of the 138 countries with comparable data, only 42 have expanded service coverage while reducing the number of people facing catastrophic OOP health spending. The number of people facing extremely high OOP health expenses has been steadily increasing worldwide. In 2019, over 1 billion people globally faced catastrophic health spending, while at the relative poverty line, the number exceeded 300 million. The number of people facing catastrophic health spend-ing increased from 588 million in 2000 to 1.04 billion in 2019, with an average annual increase of 24 million people (World Health Organization (WHO), 2023) (Figure 12.2).

OOP spending limits the ability of households to afford essential goods and services like food, shelter, clothing and education. The percentage of people living in households where more than 10% of the budget is spent on OOP health expenses has also been rising. It went from 9.6% in 2000 to 13.5% in 2019. In terms of demographics, older individuals are more likely to experience these high expenses within countries. Interestingly, there is no clear correlation between a country's income level and the rates of these OOP health expenses (World Health Organization (WHO), 2023).

Financial hardship is mostly concentrated among households with lower income due to higher rates of impoverishing health spending. In 2019, the esti-mated total population experiencing catastrophic or impoverishing health spend-ing, or both, was 2 billion people. Data shows that within countries, households with lower income were more likely to experience financial hardship. Among

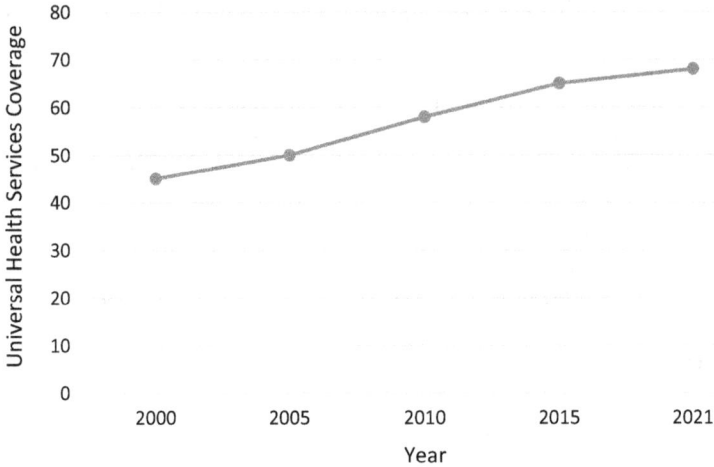

Figure 12.2 Trends in the incidence of impoverishing OOP health spending at the extreme and relative poverty lines, 2000–2019

countries, impoverishing OOP health spending at the extreme poverty line is mainly concentrated in low-income and middle-income countries with higher poverty rates. Middle-income countries experienced the largest increase in the proportion of the population facing impoverishing health spending at the relative poverty line (World Health Organization (WHO), 2023).

Catastrophic health spending: In the two decades leading up to the COVID-19 pandemic, the percentage of people globally experiencing catastrophic health spending, which is defined as spending over 10% of their household budget on health expenses, increased from 9.6% in 2000 to 12.6% in 2015 and reached 13.5% in 2019. On the other hand, the proportion of the global population pushed into poverty or further impoverished due to OOP health spending decreased from 22.2% in 2000 to 15.6% in 2015 and 4.4% in 2019 when measured against the extreme poverty line. However, the portion of the population pushed into poverty or further impoverished when measured against the relative poverty line increased from 11.8% in 2000 to 15.6% in 2015 and 16.7% in 2019.

Only a small percentage of people experience both catastrophic and impoverishing health spending simultaneously, with 12.6% facing relative poverty and 8.6% facing extreme poverty due to health expenses during the 2010–2019 period. In total, between 1.3 and 2 billion people globally experienced financial hardship in 2019, including 1 billion facing catastrophic health spending and 344 million facing impoverishing health spending at the extreme poverty line. Financial hardship is more common among poorer households due to higher rates of impoverishing health spending rather than catastrophic health spending. The occurrence of catastrophic and impoverishing health spending also varies according to other sociodemographic characteristics of households (World Health Organization (WHO), 2023).

The proportion of the global population facing catastrophic OOP health spending at thresholds of 10% and 25% continuously increased from 2000 to reach 13.5% and 3.8%, respectively, in 2019. The proportion of the population spending more than 10% of their household budget on health expenses increased from 9.6% in 2000 to 15.6% in 2015 and 13.5% in 2019, with an average annual increase of 0.2 percentage points. Similarly, the proportion using more than 25% of their household budget on OOP health spending rose from 1.9% in 2000 to 3.3% in 2015 and 3.8% in 2019, with an average annual increase of 0.1 percentage points. The annual increase in catastrophic health spending at both thresholds remained consistent before and after 2015, with an increase of 0.1 percentage points for the 10% threshold and 0.2 percentage points for the 25% threshold (World Health Organization (WHO), 2023).

The rise in catastrophic health spending is consistent with the fact that people are allocating a larger portion of their increasing consumption towards OOP health expenses. This increase in catastrophic spending occurred alongside a global increase in private consumption levels. In 88 out of 176 countries with available data, the proportion of OOP health spending in total private consumption increased from 2000 to 2019, partially explaining the global increase in catastrophic health spending. While this suggests that people are spending more on health and potentially receiving more care, reliance on OOP spending prevents higher incomes from translating into improved welfare. This highlights a global failure to efficiently utilise additional resources through pre-payment mechanisms that distribute and pool funds, unlike OOP health spending (World Health Organization (WHO), 2023).

Impoverishing health spending: The proportion of the global population facing impoverishing OOP health spending has significantly decreased for those living in extreme poverty while it has increased for those in relative poverty. The number of people impoverished or further impoverished at the extreme poverty line reduced by an average of 74 million per year, but still represented almost half of the global population living in extreme poverty in 2019. At the relative poverty line, the number of people with impoverishing health spending increased by 31 million per year, reaching almost 1.3 billion people. Any amount of OOP health spending can be a burden for people in poverty or near poverty, even if it is less than 10% of their household budget (World Health Organization (WHO), 2023).

The share of the population facing impoverishing OOP health spending at the extreme poverty line has decreased, but there has been an increase for those in relative poverty. The percentage of the population with impoverishing OOP health spending at the extreme poverty line decreased by 80%, from 22.2% in 2000 to 4.4% in 2019, while the percentage at the relative poverty line increased by 42%, from 11.8% to 16.7% during the same period. While the overall poverty levels decreased, those affected by impoverishing OOP health spending were still concentrated among the poorer segments of society (World Health Organization (WHO), 2023). Between 2015 and 2019, the incidence of impoverishing OOP health spending at the extreme poverty line reduced at a rate of 0.9 percentage points per year, while the incidence at the relative poverty line increased at a rate of 0.3 percentage points per year. This implies that health systems lack sufficient financial protection for those living in or near poverty. Over the past two decades, OOP health spending has hindered global poverty eradication efforts (World Health Organization (WHO), 2023).

Country-level progress and challenges towards universal health coverage

Countries around the world are in varying stages of progress towards UHC. There are countries which have been successful in their efforts towards UHC. Countries vary significantly in their routes towards UHC; these have been framed by particular moral claims and world views and shaped by prominent leaders and strong popular movements. Countries reach UHC at different income levels and with different institutional arrangements. Despite the substantial differences in income, political regimes, cultures and health sector institutions, countries with UHC share commonalities, including widespread and persistent domestic pressures, large role for government, emerging from negotiation rather than design and incremental and over long periods of time. Countries aspiring for UHC should thus pay attention to these commonalities (Savedoff & Smith, 2011). Analysis of nine low-income and lower-middle-income countries in Africa and Asia that have implemented national health insurance reforms towards UHC indicated that there were some trends in these countries' progress towards UHC, such as increasing enrolment in government health insurance, a movement towards expanded benefits packages, and decreasing OOP spending accompanied by increasing government share of spending on health (Lagomarsino et al., 2012).

On the other hand, there are other low- and middle-income countries which face challenges in their endeavours towards UHC. These challenges include lack of fiscal space, high donor dependence, under-developed pre-payment systems and the inadequate health systems (Jabeen et al., 2021). Shortages in human resources and medical supplies, socio-cultural barriers, physical inaccessibility, lack of education and information, decision-making power, and gender-based autonomy still deter access to, and use of, health services in these countries (Fantaye & Yaya, 2019).

A systematic review on health financing towards achieving UHC in the Southeast Asian region identified six challenges: (1) unsustainability of revenue-raising methods, (2) fragmented health insurance schemes, (3) incongruity between insurance benefits and people's needs, (4) political and legislative indifference, (5) intractable and rapidly rising healthcare cost, (6) morally reprehensible behaviours (Lim et al., 2023). The experiences of different countries show that health insurance-based models, either social or private, are not as satisfactory as public, universal health systems (Giovanella et al., 2018). Malaysia, Thailand and Singapore have achieved UHC by gradually increasing allocation for health and through various mechanisms, such as health insurance schemes which covered different segments of the population, and partnerships with private-sector providers (Jabeen et al., 2021). Malaysia has made substantial progress in providing access to healthcare for its citizens. The country's healthcare coverage and outcomes are approaching levels achieved by high-income countries (Rannan-Eliya et al., 2016).

Thailand has adopted a progressive approach towards UHC. Since the 1970s, Thailand's health development has focused on investment in the health delivery infrastructure at the district level (including community health programmes) and on training the health workforce. Targeted insurance schemes for different population groups have been implemented since 1975 and have improved financial access to healthcare until UHC was launched in 2002. Thai's government made a bold decision to use general taxation to finance its universal coverage scheme despite its low gross national income per capita. As a result, there has been a substantial reduction in levels of OOP payments, incidence of catastrophic health spending, and medical impoverishment, as well as gaps in child mortality and other health outcomes (Tangcharoensathien et al., 2018).

Thailand's exemplary success is possible through a tax-financed scheme, a comprehensive benefit package and gradual extension of coverage to illnesses that can lead to catastrophic expenditure, and capacity to mobilise adequate resources. The lessons from Thailand demonstrate the importance of continued political support, evidence informed decisions, and a capable purchaser organisation. A well-designed strategic purchasing approach has contributed to efficiency, cost containment and equity in the country. The purchaser-provider split has enabled the country to enforce accountability (Tangcharoensathien et al., 2015). This is facilitated by continued political and financial commitments to the scheme despite political rivalry (Tangcharoensathien et al., 2013).

The well-founded healthcare delivery system and favourable benefits package concertedly support the achievement of UHC goals of access and financial risk protection. Using the 10% threshold, the incidence of catastrophic spending dropped from 6.0% in 1996 to 2% in 2015. The incidence of impoverishment against the national poverty line reduced considerably from 2.2% in 1996 to approximately 0.3% in 2015. When the international poverty line of US$ 3.1 per capita per day was applied, the incidence of impoverishment was 1.4% and 0.4% in 1996 and 2015 respectively (Tangcharoensathien, Tisayaticom, et al., 2020).

Vietnam expanded its UHC gradually by prioritising the poor in an incremental way and providing a comprehensive and universal service packages thereby approaching UHC in a more equitable manner. Political commitment, sustainable financial sources and administrative capacity are strong driving factors in achieving UHC through health insurance reform (Mao et al., 2020). Similarly, Indonesia launched a comprehensive health insurance scheme in January 2014. It has implemented various health insurance schemes targeted towards the poor and near-poor, including the Jamkesmas programme. Poor women with Jamkesmas membership had a modest increase in health facility delivery and skilled birth attendance, consistent with economic theory that health insurance coverage can reduce financial barriers to care and increase service uptake. However, there are limitations in several factors, such as socio-cultural beliefs, accessibility and quality of care, which are important elements towards UHC (Brooks et al., 2017). Indonesia's journey towards UHC has been determined largely by politics. UHC became possible when the interests of politically and economically influential groups were satisfied. Access to healthcare increased as socio-economic and political importance grew (Pisani et al., 2017).

Four lessons could be learned from the Indonesian experience of developing and launching national social health insurance: the importance of strong political commitment; the role of comprehensive analysis of the national health system; the use of multiparty participation in developing and implementing the plans; and the importance of systematic, continuous monitoring and evaluation from technical and administrative perspectives as well as patient satisfaction, to assure progress towards UHC (Mboi, 2015). The UHC system grew rapidly and covers 203 million people, the largest single-payer scheme in the world, and has improved health equity and service access (Agustina et al., 2019). Insurance coverage is highest in poorer areas, where service provision, and thus service use and health spending, are lowest. The Indonesian public insurance system protects many inpatients, especially the poorest, from excessive spending (Pratiwi et al., 2021).

Bangladesh introduced a comprehensive set of policies for UHC, and has made progress in a number of areas including the roll out of the essential package of health services for all, and expansion of access to PHC services. Even though there is a strong political commitment, there are barriers due to a rigid public financing system, health system weaknesses, socio-cultural and economic challenges, mistrust and lack of community empowerment (Joarder et al., 2019). In Myanmar, attainment of UHC is challenged by low health service coverage, high financial risk and inequalities in access to care. It is recommended that health service coverage and financial risk protection for vulnerable, disadvantaged populations should be prioritised (Han et al., 2018).

Latin American countries are also advancing towards UHC. There are lessons on the separation of the three main functions of health systems: financing, delivery and stewardship in Latin American countries. Countries in the region introduced social sector reforms, underpinned by the principles of equity, solidarity and collective action to overcome social inequalities, to alleviate poverty, reduce socio-economic inequalities, improve health outcomes and provide financial risk protection since the late 1980s. There have also been health systems strengthening reforms to reduce inequalities in health access and outcomes through UHC with a special focus to poor citizens since the 1990s (Frenk & Gómez-Dantés, 2018).

Tax-financed universal health systems were introduced in countries, such as Brazil and Cuba. These financing systems enabled the introduction of supply-side interventions to expand insurance coverage, with defined and enlarged benefits packages, and to scale-up delivery of health services. These changes were combined with demand-side interventions targeting social determinants of health and improving access of disadvantaged populations (Atun et al., 2015).

Peru has implemented a progressive path towards UHC to reduce inequalities in access to healthcare by granting the poor entitlement to tax-financed basic care without charge. Consequently, the probability of receiving healthcare increased by almost two-fifths, while the inability to afford treatment reduced by more than a quarter. However, there is no effect on average OOP spending (Neelsen & O'Donnell, 2017). Haiti also faces challenges, including geographic access, financial coverage and service access. These challenges are, in turn, due to unstable financing mechanisms, including inappropriate resource allocation and ineffective management (Hashimoto et al., 2020).

In sub-Saharan Africa (SSA), direct OOP payments in many countries accounted for an average of 36% of current health expenditure compared to only 22% in the rest of the world. There is a growing recognition of the need to reduce OOP payments and increase domestic mandatory pre-payment financing to move towards UHC. Many SSA countries have declared a preference for achieving this through contributory health insurance schemes, particularly for formal sector workers, with service entitlements tied to contributions (McIntyre et al., 2018).

A review of UHC in Ghana, Kenya, Nigeria and Tanzania identified several challenges, including extreme poverty and unable to pay premiums, large informal sector employees whose members are mostly uninsured, high dropout rate from insurance schemes, poorly funded PHC system, and segmented health insurance, for UHC (Umeh, 2018). More specifically, the National Health Insurance Scheme in Ghana reported challenges that include: cost escalation, political interference, inadequate technical capacity, spatial distribution of health facilities and health workers, inadequate monitoring mechanisms, broad benefits package, large exemption groups, inadequate client education and limited community engagement (Alhassan et al., 2016). Therefore, it will be important for these countries to: (1) raise sufficient revenue to finance their health systems; (2) improve the efficiency of revenue utilisation; (3) identify and provide coverage for the very poor; (4) reduce the proportion of the population that is under-insured and (5) improve access to quality healthcare in rural areas (Umeh, 2018).

Ethiopia has recorded impressive progress towards UHC. This has been possible through its pro-poor health policy and successive strategies, including health systems strengthening, disease control programmes as well as improvements in social determinants of health (Habtemariam & Semegn, 2018). Despite these overall successes, key challenges remain: inadequate coverage, inequity, slow health systems transition to provide services for non-communicable diseases, high OOP expenditure, and inadequate quality of care. These persistent and emerging challenges are due to limitations in the health system as well as inadequacy and inequities in socio-economic conditions of populations and locations. The aspiration for health and well-being requires the country to do more and better. It is imperative that the country strengthens its health system further, integrate disease control programmes and improve multisectoral actions (Assefa, Hill, Gilks, Admassu, et al., 2020). It is commendable that the country has included equity and quality as its key transformation agendas towards UHC (Mullan, 2016).

In Rwanda, solidarity support for the poor and good connection between local leaders and heads of health facilities were identified as enablers of health service utilisation. On the other hand, shortages of skilled health providers, sparsely distributed health infrastructure, and hilly topography as well as muddy roads were identified as barriers to access health services and poor maternal health outcomes (Sayinzoga et al., 2019). Overall, effective strategies to increase access to health services and improve health status include both supply side interventions (such as delivery of services at or closer to home and service level improvements, such as integration of services) as well as demand side interventions (such as educational programmes, text messages and financial or other incentives) (Bright et al., 2017).

Pivotal in setting Rwanda on the path to UHC is the community-based health insurance (CBHI), which covers more than three-quarters of the population. Rwanda is the country with the highest enrolment in health insurance in SSA. The commitment to expanding health insurance coverage was made possible by a dominant political settlement. CBHI is part of the broader efforts of the regime to foster its legitimacy based on rapid socio-economic development (Chemouni, 2018; Nyandekwe et al., 2014).

Nigeria faces challenges that delay progress towards the attainment of UHC. One such challenge is inequities resulting from lack of financial protection. Nigeria's experience shows that where political leaders are interested in a UHC-related proposal, the strong political leadership they provide considerably enhances the pace of the policy process. The most successful period of the policy process for the inclusion of Health Maintenance Organizations (HMOs), as financing organisations for national health insurance, occurred when a new minister of health (strongly supported by the president who displayed interest in UHC) provided leadership, and effectively managed stakeholders' interests and galvanised their support to advance the policy. In contexts where authority is shared between federal and state governments, securing federal level commitment with an active role of states in the process and governance structure is crucial (Onoka et al., 2015). It is vital to encourage the states to establish and manage their own insurance funds while encouraging integration with the National Health Insurance Scheme (Okpani & Abimbola, 2015).

In Malawi, gaps in financial protection are mainly triggered by supply-side access-related barriers in the public health sector, including shortages of medicines, emergency services, shortage of health personnel and facilities, poor health workers' attitudes, distance and transportation difficulties, and perceived poor quality of health services. Moving towards UHC in Malawi requires the introduction of appropriate interventions to fill the financial protection gaps in the private sector and the access-related gaps in the public sector as well as an effective public-private partnership that completely integrates both sectors (Abiiro et al., 2014).

The SARS-Cov-2/COVID-19 pandemic affects progress towards universal health coverage

The COVID-19 pandemic had a negative impact on the progress of countries towards UHC, with no change in the global UHC index score between 2019 and 2021. While there were sub-regional and country-level decreases in some dimensions of the UHC index, the global index remained stagnant. The impact of the COVID-19 pandemic on UHSC was varied across different levels – global, regional and country. Disruptions in health services due to COVID-19 were caused by a combination of demand and supply factors, as well as the allocation of health system resources to COVID-19-related services. The pandemic's impact on the economy, fiscal situation and health led to a weakening of financial protection globally, resulting in more people facing financial hardship and forgoing care due to financial barriers. The COVID-19 pandemic has further exposed inequities and disrupted essential health services.

The COVID-19 pandemic highlights the importance of resilient health systems and public investment in primary and hospital care. UHSC needs to be prioritised for emergency preparedness. Strong public investment in PHC and health systems is crucial (World Health Organization (WHO), 2023). The COVID-19 pandemic proves that investing on health systems towards UHC and health for all is not optional (Hussain & Arif, 2021). Universal health coverage affects how a country is able to prevent, detect or respond to an infectious disease outbreak. Low or no financial barriers in accessing health services facilitate early case detection, identification of contacts. It protects people from catastrophic health expenditure and impoverishment, which further contributes to spread of the epidemic.

The COVID-19 pandemic confirms the necessity of a comprehensive and inclusive UHC (Armocida et al., 2020). Initiatives to move towards UHC must integrate global health security and health system strengthening (Jain & Alam, 2017). It is essential to build a resilient health system to improve health security

(Kruk et al., 2015). This requires higher investments to strengthen community health programmes, surveillance and emergency preparedness. This needs a strong political commitment with a vision of a more sustainable system and resilient society (Armocida et al., 2020).

Financing to achieve universal health coverage

Country commitments to UHC have increased over time. However, there is inadequate financing for health, which has impeded progress towards UHC by 2030. Although many countries have adopted UHC laws and included it in their health plans, few have clear action plans or roadmaps. Current investment commitments and public spending for health are insufficient to achieve UHC. There is over reliance on OOP payments (Nde et al., 2019). Vulnerable groups still face financial barriers to accessing healthcare. While there are existing policies to reduce these barriers, they are not reaching those in need (World Health Organization (WHO), 2023). Moreover, there is a reliance on disease-specific programmes instead of comprehensive UHC commitments. Efforts to implement disease-specific programmes, largely communicable, outnumber those for PHC and comprehensive programmes. While there is recognition of the need for comprehensive healthcare and health systems strengthening, only a small percentage of countries prioritise these in their UHC commitments (World Health Organization (WHO), 2023).

Financial protection systems should address the challenges of people forgoing care due to financial barriers. Data before the COVID-19 pandemic revealed that 19% of individuals in low- and middle-income countries reported facing financial barriers and forgoing needed care. Apart from catastrophic and impoverishing OOP spending, financial protection systems should enable access to necessary healthcare. Pre-paid pooled contributions to healthcare should be encouraged, and OOP health spending should be minimised for those living close to poverty and exempted for those living in poverty (Wang et al., 2018b). Efforts should be made to decrease financial hardship by increasing public health funding, improving efficiency and equity in healthcare, extending coverage for medicines, and implementing low, fixed and capped co-payments for those who still need and able to pay, while completely removing payments for the poor and vulnerable (World Health Organization (WHO), 2023).

There is a limited number of countries with effective accountability mechanisms for UHC. Non-state actors are inadequately engaged in these mechanisms. Populations are often passive recipients rather than active stakeholders in UHC. There is also a lack of detailed information on health expenditures. It often focuses on disease-specific programmes and lack attention to service coverage and financial protection indicators. A well-developed and comprehensive national health expenditure data system is, thus, essential in collecting, compiling and making use of data for policy-making and appropriate investment (World Health Organization (WHO), 2023).

13 The public health approaches towards universal health coverage

A successful public health approach in the HIV/AIDS response

Public health functions are the set of actions that are fundamental for achieving the goal of public health, which is to improve, promote, protect and restore the health of the population, through collective action (World Health Organization (WHO), 2018a). Public health approaches are, thus, comprehensive strategies that aim to improve population health and well-being by implementing population-level policies that promote healthy behaviours, prevent diseases and address social determinants of health. They promote healthy lifestyles through education and awareness campaigns as well as immunisation programmes, screening, and early detection and treatment. They can also significantly reduce the burden on healthcare systems and improve overall population health by preventing diseases (Shi et al., 2009).

They involve a range of strategies and policies that target various levels of society, from individuals to communities and entire populations (Shi et al., 2009). These strategies and policies recognise the impact of social determinants of health including factors such as socio-economic status, education, employment and access to healthcare. By addressing social determinants of health, public health approaches aim to reduce health disparities and improve health equity (Thornton et al., 2016).

Different communities have unique health needs and challenges, and public health approaches aim to address these differences through culturally sensitive and inclusive strategies. This involves engaging with communities, understanding their perspectives and needs, and involving them in the decision-making process (Gillies, 1998).

Public health approaches also emphasise the importance of surveillance and monitoring, which involve collecting and analysing data on health outcomes, risk factors and health behaviours to inform decision-making and evaluate effectiveness of interventions (Cameron et al., 2007). Monitoring, evaluation and continuous improvement are integral to public health approaches to ensure that resources are allocated efficiently and that interventions are achieving their intended outcomes (Choi, 2012; Remington & Nelson, 2010).

DOI: 10.4324/9781003505693-17

Public health approaches have played a crucial role in HIV/AIDS prevention and control efforts by focusing on prevention, testing, care, addressing social determinants, harm reduction, community engagement, integration, surveillance, international collaboration and research. These approaches contribute to reducing the impact of HIV/AIDS on individuals and communities, ultimately working towards the goal of ending the epidemic. They encompass a range of strategies aimed at addressing the social and structural factors to reduce the transmission of HIV and improve access to treatment and care (Ford et al., 2018; Gilks et al., 2006).

Public health approaches recognise the global nature of the HIV/AIDS epidemic and the need for international collaboration. Through partnerships with international organisations, governments and donors, public health efforts can leverage resources, share best practices and coordinate efforts to achieve common goals. This collaboration has been essential for advocating for policies that support HIV/AIDS control, scaling up prevention and treatment services, and strengthening health systems (Bekker et al., 2018; Piot et al., 2015).

Public health approaches for universal health coverage

Public health approaches are essential towards ensuring that everyone has access to quality healthcare services without facing financial hardship. By implementing primary healthcare, promoting health and preventing diseases, strengthening health systems, and addressing the needs of vulnerable populations, countries can move closer to achieving universal health coverage (UHC) and improving the health and well-being of their populations (Knaul et al., 2015; White, 2015).

Implementation of primary healthcare systems involves establishing a network of community-based healthcare facilities that provide essential healthcare services, including health promotion, disease prevention and treatment of common illnesses. By strengthening primary healthcare, individuals can receive timely and cost-effective care, reducing the burden on more specialised and expensive healthcare services. By empowering individuals with knowledge and skills to make informed decisions about their health, these programmes contribute to reducing the burden of preventable diseases and promoting overall well-being (De Maeseneer et al., 2020; Sacks et al., 2020; World Health Organization (WHO), 2018f).

Health promotion and disease prevention encompasses a range of strategies and interventions aimed at promoting healthy behaviours, preventing diseases and improving overall population health. It contributes to creating a healthier population and a more equitable healthcare system by addressing the underlying determinants of health, empowering individuals and communities, and advocating for policies that promote health and well-being (Oni et al., 2019). It empowers individuals to make informed decisions about their health by providing them with the necessary knowledge and skills (Epp, 1986). Through education campaigns and awareness programmes, people can adopt healthier lifestyles, engage in risk-reduction behaviours and actively participate in managing their health (Coe & de Beyer, 2014; Shilton & Barry, 2022). It also focuses on preventive measures, such as immunisations, which can significantly reduce the burden of diseases. It also contributes to reducing healthcare costs and ensuring that resources are allocated efficiently within the framework of UHC (Woolf et al., 2008). It enables prompt treatment and management by encouraging regular health check-ups and screenings (Lantz et al., 2001).

It helps create a supportive environment for individuals to lead healthier lives, ultimately contributing to UHC, by advocating for policies that tackle these underlying factors (Brennan Ramirez et al., 2008). It supports the development of healthy public policies that promote health and well-being, such as tobacco control measures, healthy food environments and safe working conditions (Jackson et al., 2006; World Health Organization (WHO), 1986). It recognises the intersectoral nature of health and collaborates with various sectors, including education, transportation and urban planning. By integrating health considerations into policies and practices across sectors, health promotion helps create environments that promote health and reduce health inequities, a key objective of UHC (Corbin, 2017).

Health promotion ensures that interventions are culturally appropriate, relevant and sustainable by involving communities in the planning, implementation and evaluation of health programmes. This is essential for achieving UHC, as it promotes inclusivity and equity in healthcare delivery (Haldane et al., 2019). By promoting equitable access to healthcare, health promotion contributes to reducing health inequalities and ensuring that no one is left behind in the pursuit of UHC (El Ansari et al., 2009).

Primary prevention reduces the demand for curative services, allowing healthcare systems to allocate resources more efficiently. It also promotes integrated and people-centred care, fostering a holistic approach to health that aligns with the principles of UHC (Van den Broucke, 2017). Investing in primary prevention is not only cost-effective but also leads to long-term health benefits. By promoting health and preventing diseases, healthcare systems can allocate resources more efficiently and focus on providing necessary care for those who need it the most (World Health Organization (WHO), 2005a).

Secondary prevention is a crucial component of UHC, aiming to detect and treat diseases at an early stage to prevent their progression and minimise their impact on individuals and communities. By implementing effective secondary prevention strategies, healthcare systems can improve health outcomes, reduce healthcare costs and enhance overall population health (Niessen & Squire, 2019). Timely diagnosis is crucial for effective treatment and management of diseases. This helps prevent complications, manage chronic conditions and improve overall health outcomes. Care and treatment services should aim to provide integrated healthcare by coordinating different healthcare providers and services. This ensures that individuals receive comprehensive and coordinated care, reducing fragmentation and improving the overall quality of care (Mazaba et al., 2016; Samuel et al., 2020).

Care and treatment services also encompass palliative care, which focuses on improving the quality of life for individuals with serious illnesses. Palliative care addresses physical, emotional and psychosocial needs of patients and their families (Bates et al., 2019; Knaul et al., 2019).

Health system strengthening and governance for universal health coverage

Health system strengthening involves improving the capacity and efficiency of healthcare systems, including healthcare workforce development, infrastructure development and health information systems. By strengthening the overall health system, countries can provide comprehensive and integrated healthcare services to their populations (Jaca et al., 2022; Kieny et al., 2017).

Effective governance is essential for the efficient and equitable delivery of healthcare services towards UHC. It involves the structures, processes and mechanisms through which health policies are formulated, implemented and monitored (Yeoh et al., 2019). It encompasses policy formulation, stakeholder participation, capacity building, financing, monitoring, equity, patient-centred care and international cooperation. These policies should address issues such as healthcare financing, service delivery, human resources and quality assurance. Governance ensures that healthcare services are provided in a standardised and consistent manner across the country (Hort et al., 2017). By strengthening governance mechanisms, countries can thus ensure the provision of accessible, affordable and high-quality healthcare services for all (Debie et al., 2022).

It focuses on strengthening the capacity of healthcare institutions and professionals. By investing in the development of the workforce, governance ensures the provision of high-quality and accessible healthcare services (Jaca et al., 2022). It plays a crucial role in healthcare financing. It involves innovative financing models, such as social health insurance or taxation, to generate funds for healthcare services. It ensures that financial resources are utilised efficiently and equitably (Afriyie et al., 2021).

Health systems governance promotes the integration of health services across different levels of care. It encourages coordination and collaboration among primary care providers, hospitals and specialised healthcare facilities. This ensures that individuals receive comprehensive and continuous care (Tumusiime et al., 2019). It also promotes patient-centred care by emphasising the importance of patient rights, dignity and participation in decision-making processes and protection of their privacy (Lewis & Pettersson Gelander, 2009). It plays a crucial role in ensuring equity in healthcare delivery by addressing social determinants of health and promoting equal access to healthcare services (Siddiqi et al., 2009).

Health systems governance fosters innovation and the adoption of new technologies in healthcare. By embracing innovation, governance ensures that healthcare systems keep pace with advancements in medical science and technology (Balasubramaniam et al., 2018). By monitoring performance indicators, governance enables evidence-based decision-making and facilitates continuous quality improvement in healthcare services (Arhin et al., 2023).

It ensures the participation of various stakeholders in decision-making processes. This promotes transparency, accountability and responsiveness in healthcare decision-making (Paolucci et al., 2017). It also plays a crucial role in fostering global health partnerships, sharing best practices and learning from experiences of other countries (Robert et al., 2022).

Health services delivery for universal health coverage

Countries can move closer to achieving UHC through a comprehensive, equitable, quality-focused, financially sustainable and patient-centred approach (Bloom, 2019; Fusheini & Eyles, 2016). It should promote health promotion and disease prevention, including public health interventions, such as immunisation programmes, health education campaigns and screening services (Shilton & Barry, 2022). This should be based on a strong primary healthcare system that acts as the first point of contact for individuals seeking healthcare (Whiting et al., 2016). It should prioritise equity and address the needs of vulnerable populations. Efforts should be made to reduce health disparities and ensure that marginalised groups have equal access to healthcare services (Macdonald et al., 2019; Rao et al., 2019). It should also be responsive to the evolving health needs of the population. Health providers should be well-trained, competent and adhere to ethical standards to ensure the delivery of high-quality care (Ehrenkranz et al., 2021).

Differentiated service delivery models for universal health coverage: Differentiated service delivery models are innovative approaches that aim to provide equitable and accessible healthcare services to all individuals, regardless of their socio-economic status or geographical location. These models recognise that different populations have diverse healthcare needs and require tailored interventions to ensure optimal health outcomes. These models encompass a range of approaches, including task-shifting, specialised clinics, mHealth, community-based health insurance, integrated care, telemedicine, pharmaceutical care, school-based health programmes and community health worker programmes. By implementing differentiated service delivery models, countries can enhance the effectiveness and efficiency of their healthcare systems, ultimately contributing to the achievement of UHC goals, including improved health outcomes and a more inclusive healthcare system (Ehrenkranz et al., 2021).

Integration towards universal health coverage: Integration of services plays a crucial role in achieving UHC. This integration involves bringing together different healthcare providers, facilities and programmes to provide comprehensive and coordinated care that can enhance efficiency, effectiveness and equity (Lê et al., 2016). Integrating services across different levels of care is crucial for UHC (R. Khatri et al., 2023). This involves linking primary, secondary and tertiary care facilities to ensure a seamless flow of patients and information. By establishing referral systems and strengthening the linkages between primary care providers and specialised healthcare facilities, individuals can receive timely and appropriate care, reducing the need for costly and unnecessary referrals (Mendes & Almeida, 2020). This integration also promotes continuity of care, ensuring that individuals receive comprehensive and holistic healthcare services (Tan & Earn Lee, 2019).

Integrating preventive and promotive services is essential for achieving UHC (World Health Organization (WHO), 2018d). By incorporating preventive measures such as vaccinations, screenings and health education into routine healthcare services, it is possible to prevent the onset of diseases and promote healthy behaviours. This not only improves health outcomes but also reduces the burden on healthcare systems by preventing the progression of diseases to more advanced stages (Gröne & Garcia-Barbero, 2001).

Furthermore, integration of health information systems, through implementation of electronic health records and interoperable systems, improves care coordination, reduces duplication of services and enhances patient safety by ensuring that healthcare providers have access to complete and accurate medical histories (Asah & Nielsen, 2016; Tossy, 2014).

Integration also involves engaging communities and empowering individuals to actively participate in their healthcare. This integration promotes community ownership and accountability, leading to improved health outcomes and increased satisfaction with healthcare services (Chen et al., 2016; Rifkin, 2003). Moreover, integrating social determinants of health into healthcare systems is crucial for achieving UHC. This involves collaborating with other sectors, such as education, housing and social welfare, to create a comprehensive approach to health that goes beyond the traditional healthcare setting (Gurewich et al., 2020; Russell et al., 2013).

The integration of financing mechanisms is essential for UHC. By pooling resources and implementing risk-sharing mechanisms, healthcare systems can ensure that everyone has access to needed services without facing financial hardship. This integration involves aligning different financing schemes to create a sustainable and equitable healthcare financing system (Myint et al., 2019).

Integrating technology and innovation into healthcare systems can enhance service delivery and improve access to care. Individuals can access healthcare services remotely by leveraging digital health solutions, telemedicine and mobile health applications (Lygidakis et al., 2016). This integration also enables the collection and analysis of health data, leading to evidence-based decision-making and improved health outcomes (Hussein, 2015; Thakur et al., 2012).

Decentralisation of services towards universal health coverage: Decentralisation of services plays a vital role in achieving UHC. One of the key benefits of decentralisation is improved accessibility to healthcare services by bringing healthcare services closer to the communities (Abimbola et al., 2019). It improves accessibility, promotes community engagement, enhances efficiency and fosters equity in healthcare provision (Cobos Muñoz et al., 2017). It distributes the burden of healthcare provision across various levels of government and healthcare facilities, allowing for more efficient and equitable delivery of healthcare (Ati, 2018; Okech, 2017). Decentralisation enables tailored and responsive healthcare services that meet the diverse needs of communities by empowering local authorities and healthcare facilities. This is particularly important for individuals residing in remote or underserved areas (Bossert, 2013; Okech, 2017).

Decentralisation also fosters equity in healthcare provision. By bringing services closer to the communities, marginalised and vulnerable populations, such as those living in poverty, are more likely to receive the care they need. This helps address existing health disparities and ensures that no one is left behind in the pursuit of UHC. Additionally, decentralisation allows for the tailoring of healthcare services to specific population groups, taking into account their cultural, social and linguistic needs (Alves et al., 2013).

However, it is important to note that decentralisation also presents challenges that need to be addressed (Atkinson & Haran, 2004). Effective coordination and collaboration between different levels of government and healthcare facilities is crucial to ensure seamless service delivery. Adequate funding and resource allocation mechanisms must be in place to support decentralised healthcare systems. Moreover, capacity building efforts are necessary to empower local authorities and healthcare professionals with the skills and knowledge required to effectively manage and deliver healthcare services (Dick-Sagoe, 2020; Dwicaksono & Fox, 2018).

Health systems financing for universal health coverage

Health systems financing plays a crucial role in achieving UHC, which aims to ensure that all individuals and communities have access to quality health services without suffering financial hardship. It involves the mobilisation, pooling, allocation and utilisation of funds to provide services, develop infrastructure and build health workforce capacity (Kutzin, 2013).

A robust and efficient health financing mechanism should be designed to pool resources from various sources, such as government revenues, social health insurance contributions, and external aid, to create a sustainable funding pool, which will be shared among the population, reducing the risk of catastrophic health expenditures for individuals and households (Mathauer et al., 2020). By investing in robust health financing mechanisms, countries can move closer to achieving UHC and ensuring that everyone has access to the healthcare they need without financial hardship (Kutzin, 2013).

Sustainable health systems financing involves strategic planning and forecasting to anticipate future health needs and allocate resources accordingly. This includes investing in health infrastructure, technology and human resources to meet the evolving healthcare demands of the population (Thomson et al., 2009). Innovative financing mechanisms, such as public-private partnerships or health insurance schemes, can help diversify funding sources and enhance financial sustainability (Liaropoulos & Goranitis, 2015).

Transparency and accountability are essential in health systems financing. Governments and health authorities should ensure that financial resources are used efficiently, effectively, and in line with national health policies and priorities. Regular financial audits and public reporting can help build trust and ensure that funds are being used for their intended purpose (Uzochukwu et al., 2018).

It is essential to invest in sectors beyond healthcare, such as education, housing and sanitation, that can have a significant impact on population health outcomes. By addressing the underlying social and economic factors that influence health, health systems financing can contribute to reducing health inequities and improving overall well-being (Bayarsaikhan et al., 2022).

Political commitment and leadership are crucial for successful financing. Governments should prioritise health as a fundamental human right and allocate sufficient resources to achieve UHC. This requires engaging stakeholders, including civil society organisations, the private sector and communities, in the decision-making process (Kelsall et al., 2016).

External aid plays a significant role in health systems financing for UHC, particularly in low-income countries with limited domestic resources. Development partners can provide financial and technical support to strengthen health systems, build capacity and bridge funding gaps. However, it is important to ensure that external aid aligns with national health priorities and is coordinated to avoid fragmentation and duplication of efforts (Zakumumpa et al., 2019).

Human resources for health towards universal health coverage

Human resources for health (HRH) play a crucial role in achieving UHC. In order to achieve UHC, it is essential to have an adequate and well-distributed workforce of skilled health workers. By investing in HRH, countries can ensure the availability, accessibility and quality of healthcare services for all individuals and communities. HRH plays a crucial role in reducing health inequities, strengthening health systems, responding to emergencies, promoting health promotion, fostering innovation, ensuring sustainability and fostering global health partnerships (Campbell et al., 2013; Haakenstad et al., 2022).

Task shifting and task sharing play crucial roles in achieving UHC by optimising the utilisation of healthcare resources and addressing the shortage of skilled healthcare professionals. These strategies involve redistributing tasks among different healthcare workers, allowing them to perform tasks that are within their scope of practice and expertise. By doing so, task shifting and task sharing enhance access to quality healthcare services, particularly in resource-constrained settings (Awolude et al., 2018; Dawson et al., 2014).

Access to essential medicines, vaccines and diagnostics for universal health coverage

Access to essential medicines, vaccines and diagnostics is a crucial aspect of achieving UHC (Adebisi et al., 2022). Access to essential medicines ensures that individuals can receive appropriate treatment and care, leading to improved health outcomes. Access to vaccines is essential to protect individuals and communities from vaccine-preventable diseases. Vaccines are crucial in preventing the spread of infectious diseases and reducing the burden on healthcare systems. Access to diagnostic tools and tests enables healthcare providers to make timely and accurate diagnosis, which is crucial for effective treatment and management of diseases (Pai & Kohli, 2019). It is, thus, essential to prioritise the availability and affordability of essential medicines, vaccines and diagnostics to ensure UHC (Bors et al., 2015).

Ensuring access to essential medicines, vaccines and diagnostics requires a comprehensive and integrated approach. It involves addressing various factors such as affordability, availability, quality and rational use of these healthcare interventions (Amimo et al., 2021). Stakeholders, including governments, private actors and international organisations, need to collaborate to develop strategies that promote equitable access to these essential health tools. Policies that promote fair pricing and reduce the financial burden on individuals and healthcare systems should be implemented. This may involve negotiating prices with pharmaceutical companies, promoting generic alternatives and implementing cost-effective procurement strategies. It is crucial to develop robust supply chains, which ensure adequate storage and distribution facilities, and provide training to healthcare workers on their appropriate use. It is also essential to promote research and development to expand the range of these essential interventions. Innovation in these areas can lead to the development of more effective and affordable healthcare interventions. International cooperation is crucial for addressing global health challenges related to access to essential medicines, vaccines and diagnostics (Chattu et al., 2023).

Health information systems for universal health coverage

Health information systems play a crucial role in achieving UHC by providing a comprehensive and efficient means of managing health data. These systems are designed to collect, store, analyse and disseminate health information, enabling healthcare providers and policymakers to make informed decisions and improve the overall quality of care. By harnessing the power of technology and data, these systems pave the way for a more equitable, efficient and sustainable healthcare system (Rashidian, 1995; Sahay et al., 2018).

One key benefit of health information systems for UHC is the ability to track and monitor population health trends. By collecting data on various health indicators such as disease prevalence, mortality rates and risk factors, these systems help identify priority areas for intervention and resource allocation. This information is essential for designing targeted healthcare programmes and policies that address the specific needs of different populations.

Furthermore, health information systems facilitate the integration and coordination of healthcare services. Through interoperable electronic health records (EHRs), healthcare providers can access and share patient information seamlessly, ensuring continuity of care across different healthcare settings. This integration not only improves patient outcomes but also reduces duplication of services and healthcare costs (Cipriano et al., 2013).

In addition, health information systems enhance the efficiency and effectiveness of healthcare delivery. By automating administrative tasks such as appointment scheduling, billing and inventory management, these systems streamline workflows and reduce the burden on healthcare professionals. This allows them to focus more on patient care and spend less time on paperwork, ultimately improving the overall quality and timeliness of healthcare services (Chaudhry et al., 2006).

Moreover, health information systems support evidence-based decision-making. By analysing large datasets, these systems generate valuable insights into healthcare outcomes, treatment effectiveness and cost-effectiveness. Policymakers can use this information to develop evidence-based policies and interventions that maximise health outcomes while optimising resource allocation (Aldhizer & Juras, 2015).

Another advantage of health information systems is their role in disease surveillance and outbreak response. By monitoring real-time data on disease incidence and spread, these systems enable early detection and rapid response to outbreaks, minimising their impact on public health. This proactive approach is essential for preventing the spread of infectious diseases and protecting the health of communities (Savel et al., 2012).

Furthermore, health information systems promote patient empowerment and engagement. Through patient portals and mobile health applications, individuals can access their own health information, track their progress and actively participate in their own care. This increased access to information and involvement in decision-making leads to better health outcomes and patient satisfaction (Rozenblum et al., 2015).

Additionally, health information systems facilitate research and innovation in healthcare. By providing researchers with access to large-scale health data, these systems support the development of new treatments, interventions and technologies. This fosters a culture of continuous improvement and drives advancements in healthcare delivery (Thakur et al., 2012). Moreover, health information systems play a vital role in monitoring and evaluating the performance of healthcare systems. By tracking key performance indicators such as wait times, patient satisfaction and healthcare utilisation, these systems help identify areas for improvement and measure the impact of interventions (Mpofu et al., 2014).

Conclusion

Our book aims to describe and analyse why globally there has been extraordinary success with HIV/AIDS control over the last two decades such that AIDS is firmly on track to end as a public health threat in most low- and middle-income jurisdictions by 2030. It then considers what lessons may be relevant for controlling the epidemic of NCDs in the global south, given the limited progress made to date. We finally consider how this can potentially drive progress towards UHC.

Starting with an explicit focus on treatment and making ART accessible to all in need, antiretroviral medicines were deployed using a WHO public health approach that effectively linked primary healthcare with hospital services in the district health team. By 2022, globally ART coverage exceeded 75% and few were falling ill with HIV-related disease or dying prematurely with AIDS. Wide availability of ARVs opened up biomedical prevention to become a mainstay of combination prevention; incidence has been steadily declining for over 20 years and HIV is now endemic in most communities.

This is in stark contrast to the limited progress made across the global south in effectively addressing the NCD epidemic, in particular implementing cost-effective best-buy policies and simple clinical interventions for their prevention and control: it is highly unlikely the SDG target to reduce by one-third premature mortality from NCDs by 2030 will be achieved. Given the parlous state of health services in resource-limited settings, significantly aggravated by SARS-CoV-2/COVID-19 pandemic, limited progress has been made with the other disease control priorities that are also major causes of disability, morbidity and premature mortality in the global south. Much needs to be done.

It seems clear that unless radical steps are taken to provide person-centred care at the PHC level and to rapidly deliver quality health services to address the full burden of disease, there is little prospect of the world making significant progress towards UHC by 2030. The UHC package includes financial risk protection, access to quality essential healthcare services and access to effective and quality affordable essential medicines and vaccines. WHO recognises that improvements to health service coverage have stagnated since 2015, and the proportion of the population facing catastrophic levels of out-of-pocket health

DOI: 10.4324/9781003505693-18

spending has increased continuously since 2000. This global pattern is consistent across all regions and the majority of countries.

Lack of progress with UHC adversely impacts global development and prosperity. Almost 100 million people are impoverished by health expenses every year: the first SDG "to end poverty in all its forms everywhere" is in peril without significant progress being made with UHC. It is a foundational investment in economic growth and human capital: without good health, adults are not productive and children are unable to go to school. There are many reasons why globally much more needs to be done to improve health service access, quality and performance. Major investments need to be made to strengthen health systems so as significantly to improve health outcomes.

These investments were made in HIV/AIDS control: HIV service coverage has massively increased; few households face catastrophic out-of-pocket expenses for HIV care and AIDS treatment. This all came on the back of an exceptional global response, new financing mechanisms and a huge increase in earmarked domestic funding and international development assistance for health, at least until the last decade when funding has flatlined. Governments and donors are prepared to invest in HIV/AIDS services because budgets can be effectively deployed through a public health approach to generate impressive results. If it can be done for HIV/AIDS then it can and must be widely replicated across low- and middle-income countries for the NCDs and other disease control priorities.

We consider that there are several lessons from HIV/AIDS control which have direct relevance for NCDs and the other main disease control priorities in low- and middle-income countries. If acted upon, these will greatly support access to affordable, quality essential health services; and by effectively reducing major morbidity and premature mortality will provide a significant level of financial risk protection. Sustainably delivered through strengthened health systems, they can significantly enhance progress towards UHC across the global south.

The first lesson is to recognise the power of activism and concerted lobbying for a clear, focussed health outcome. People living with HIV and sick with AIDS vocally demanded care and ART for all in need; and for exceptional responses, including new funding mechanisms to close the inequitable global treatment gap. Such focal mobilisation has been successful in child survival, with GAVI the only comparable Global Health Initiative to PEPFAR and the Global Fund. It has been less successful with other disease-specific challenges like TB and malaria (outside the GFATM), the rather nebulous NCD construct and the NTDs, particularly in regard to visibility and generating earmarked funding.

The second is to acknowledge WHO's courage and leadership in taking on the challenge of universal access and closing the treatment gap when most thought this too risky and impossible to achieve. The aspirational and hugely ambitious targets of 3 million on ART by the end of 2005 were not reached. But boldly moving on from a business as usual approach, the unstoppable momentum generated in "3by5" was maintained and sustained. Closing the treatment gap is now recognised as a global public health triumph. Risks sometimes have to be taken.

The third is to recognise that a prevention-only approach with affirmative policy, risk reduction and behaviour change is broadly unacceptable to communities and populations at risk; and will not succeed unless accompanied by care and support interventions for those who are already ill and beyond prevention. The UN and WHO initially committed to closing the treatment gap then when ARV medicines were broadly available quickly integrated biomedical prevention into enhanced combination prevention. Health planners and policymakers in low- and middle-income countries should recognise that it is not an either/or approach: treatment must be linked to and integrated with prevention for success in any disease control initiative.

The fourth is to adopt a WHO public health approach to disease control that focusses on population-level outcomes, simplifies and standardises intervention packages and integrates person-centred PHC with hospital care in the district health team. Initially developed to support equitable ART scale-up, then subsequently refined over two decades of implementation, it is clear that there are similar biomedical prevention and care pathways across the NCDs and many of the disease control priorities which facilitate quality improvement and integrated service delivery. To work, all need robust and functioning health services. They are predicated on capacitated health systems capable of delivering quality services: significant investment is required for health systems strengthening.

This leads into the fifth lesson to adopt an integrated and horizontal approach that moves away from vertical single disease control programmes towards health system strengthening. Success in strengthening service delivery in one exceptionally supported area like HIV/AIDS can be replicated in another priority area if new support is forthcoming, highly unlikely today given constrained finances. It will prove hugely inefficient and impractical to have several vertical programmes working side-by-side and competing for staff and resources. Facilitated by a common public health approach, it is far better to move towards integrated service delivery across the life course and to provide exceptional sustained support to strengthen health system capacity at the PHC and district hospital level.

Good healthy costs; success breeds success. The final lesson is to applaud the achievements made in HIV/AIDS control; recognise that the elements of success, particularly the public health approach, are widely applicable to NCDs and many disease control priorities; and appreciate that sustained investment can deliver successful disease outcome. Governments and donors need confidence that major investments in health, and specifically health system strengthening, will pay off in multiple ways: reduced premature mortality; more households protected from financial hardship; improved school performance; stronger economic performance and poverty reduction. Many decision-makers view health as a bottomless pit with little return on investment: it should be widely acknowledged that HIV/AIDS has shown conclusively that this is not the case.

For the lessons to be appreciated and widely applied, significant shifts in global health architecture are needed. This involves a pivot to horizontal, integrated treatment and prevention interventions that are of sufficient quality and reach to have sustained impact on disability, major morbidity and premature mortality. To be accessible, person-centred care is best delivered in the community at the primary healthcare level; but to be comprehensive and most effective needs to be integrated with specialist hospital services through a capacitated district health team.

Global Health Initiatives and influential foundations need to shift focus from specific, often donor-derived agendas to a broader approach supporting quality service coverage across the full burden of disease. Governments and global funding mechanisms need to pivot towards general health system strengthening rather than vertical disease control programmes from confidence that significant new investment in systems rather than diseases can and will pay off in the medium to long term. WHO's role in leadership must be reinforced to lead these shifts in global health architecture.

To support these major shifts, substantial changes in global health culture and public health practice will be required. Culture is generally more resistant to change than process and practice. Public health practitioners and global health experts need more positively to appreciate the clinical skills that healthcare workers have; likewise doctors and hospital specialists should recognise that prevention is often better that cure and that it compliments their clinical practice, particularly when biomedical prevention is an important component.

All need to work to avoid divisive false dichotomies: the communicable/non-communicable binary; treatment or prevention; primary health versus hospital care; vertical or horizontal approaches; my disease is more consequential than yours. All must start from the premise that communities want better health and well-being, financial protection from catastrophic OOP health expenses and relief from disability, disease and premature death. It is not a zero-sum game; consumers do not appreciate or understand these cultural distinctions and imposed binaries. As with the "3by5" initiative, not all will be enthusiastic: some may want to continue with business as usual and preserve their speciality area and safety zone. But the status quo will never progress UHC.

Implementing these lessons and adopting integrated approaches may be a lengthy process and be slow to have significant impact, particularly reducing catastrophic out-of-pocket health expenses. These necessary developments are unlikely to deliver much to the aspirational SDG goals or come close to the numerous ambitious health and related targets by 2030. However, a start can be made with a more appropriate architecture and health culture; new approaches for strengthening health systems; and additional financing stemming from confidence that this has worked for HIV/AIDS.

Whatever replaces the SDGs in 2031, health and well-being will remain an essential component of sustainable development. Universal Health Coverage will endure as a primary objective of the global health and development enterprise and continue as the principal urgent priority. With the changes and improvements we envisage, based on success in HIV/AIDS control against all the odds, there will be momentum and progress to build on. And relative optimism that something substantial can be done to improve health outcomes and alleviate poverty for the least served and most in need.

Bibliography

Section 1

Abongomera, G., Chiwaula, L., Revill, P., Mabugu, T., Tumwesige, E., Nkhata, M., . . . Chan, A. K. (2018). Patient-level benefits associated with decentralization of antiretroviral therapy services to primary health facilities in Malawi and Uganda. *International Health, 10*(1), 8–19.

Adelman, C. C. (2006). Opinion piece 23 May 2005. Let's learn from Global Health failures. *The New York Times.*

Assefa, Y., & Gilks, C. F. (2020). Ending the epidemic of HIV/AIDS by 2030: Will there be an endgame to HIV, or an endemic HIV requiring an integrated health systems response in many countries? *International Journal of Infectious Diseases, 100,* 273–277.

Ataguba, E., Birungi, C., Cunial, S., & Kavanagh, M. (2023). Income inequality and pandemics: Insights from HIV/AIDS and COVID-19. *BMJ Global Health, 8*(9), e013703.

Autenrieth, C. S., Beck, E. J., Stelzle, D., Mallouris, C., Mahy, M., & Ghys, P. (2018). Global and regional trends of people living with HIV aged 50 and over: Estimates and projections for 2000–2020. *Plos One, 13*(11), e0207005.

Barré-Sinoussi, F., Chermann, J.-C., Rey, F., Nugeyre, M. T., Chamaret, S., Gruest, J., . . . Rouzioux, C. (1983). Isolation of a T-lymphotropic retrovirus from a patient at risk for acquired immune deficiency syndrome (AIDS). *Science, 220*(4599), 868–871.

Battistella Nemes, M. I., Beaudoin, J., Conway, S., Kivumbi, G. W., Skjelmerud, A., Vogel, U., & Organization, W. H. (2006). *Evaluation of WHO's contribution to "3 by 5": Main report.* (9241594357).

Baum, F. (2007). Health for all now! Reviving the spirit of Alma Ata in the twenty-first century: An introduction to the Alma Ata declaration. *Social Medicine, 2*(1), 34–41.

Bennett, D. E., Bertagnolio, S., Sutherland, D., & Gilks, C. F. (2008). The World Health Organization's global strategy for prevention and assessment of HIV drug resistance. *Antiviral Therapy, 13*(2_suppl), 1–13.

Bert, F., Gualano, M. R., Biancone, P., Brescia, V., Camussi, E., Martorana, M., . . . Siliquini, R. (2018). Cost-effectiveness of HIV screening in high-income countries: A systematic review. *Health Policy, 122*(5), 533–547.

Bertagnolio, S., Derdelinckx, I., Parker, M., Fitzgibbon, J., Fleury, H., Peeters, M., . . . Tanuri, A. (2008). World Health Organization/HIVResNet drug resistance laboratory strategy. *Antiviral Therapy, 13*(2_suppl), 49–57.

Bongaarts, J. (2006). UNAIDS/WHO AIDS, Epidemic Update: December 2005. *Population and Development Review, 32*(1), 184–185.

Brandt, A. M. (2013). How AIDS invented global health. *New England Journal of Medicine, 368*(23), 2149–2152.

Brown, L. B., Havlir, D. V., Ayieko, J., Mwangwa, F., Owaraganise, A., Kwarisiima, D., . . . Chamie, G. (2016). High levels of retention in care with streamlined care and universal test-and-treat in East Africa. *AIDS (London, England), 30*(18), 2855.

Burke, R. M., Feasey, N., Rangaraj, A., Camps, M. R., Meintjes, G., El-Sadr, W. M., & Ford, N. (2023). Ending AIDS deaths requires improvements in clinical care for people with advanced HIV disease who are seriously ill. *The Lancet HIV, 10*(7), e482–e484

Burki, T. (2022). The replenishment of the Global Fund. *The Lancet Infectious Diseases, 22*(11), 1546–1547.

Buse, K., & Hawkes, S. (2015). Health in the sustainable development goals: Ready for a paradigm shift? *Globalization and Health, 11*(1), 1–8.

Calabrese, S. K., & Mayer, K. H. (2020). Stigma impedes HIV prevention by stifling patient–provider communication about U=U. *Journal of the International AIDS Society, 23*(7), e25559.

Celum, C., & Baeten, J. (2020). PrEP for HIV prevention: Evidence, global scale-up, and emerging options. *Cell Host & Microbe, 27*(4), 502–506.

Chanda-Kapata, P., Ntoumi, F., Kapata, N., Lungu, P., Mucheleng'anga, L. A., Chakaya, J., . . . Asogun, D. (2022). Tuberculosis, HIV/AIDS and malaria health services in sub-Saharan Africa–a situation analysis of the disruptions and impact of the COVID-19 pandemic. *International Journal of Infectious Diseases, 124*, S41–S46.

Chintu, C., Bhat, G., Walker, A., Mulenga, V., Sinyinza, F., Lishimpi, K., . . . Gillespie, S. (2004). Co-trimoxazole as prophylaxis against opportunistic infections in HIV-infected Zambian children (CHAP): A double-blind randomised placebo-controlled trial. *The Lancet, 364*(9448), 1865–1871.

Chou, L., Harrington, M., Huff, B., Jefferys, R., Syed, J., & Wingfield, C. (2009). HIV, tuberculosis, and viral hepatitis: Drugs, diagnostics, vaccines, and microbicides in development-TAG 2009 pipeline report. *HIV, tuberculosis, and viral hepatitis: Drugs, diagnostics, vaccines, and microbicides in development-TAG 2009 pipeline report.*

Clark, J. (2014). Medicalization of global health 1: Has the global health agenda become too medicalized? *Global Health Action, 7*(1), 23998. doi:10.3402/gha.v7.23998

Cohen, M. S., Chen, Y. Q., McCauley, M., Gamble, T., Hosseinipour, M. C., Kumarasamy, N., . . . Pilotto, J. H. (2016). Antiretroviral therapy for the prevention of HIV-1 transmission. *New England Journal of Medicine, 375*(9), 830–839.

Connor, E. M., Sperling, R. S., Gelber, R., Kiselev, P., Scott, G., O'sullivan, M. J., . . . Jacobson, R. L. (1994). Reduction of maternal-infant transmission of human immunodeficiency virus type 1 with zidovudine treatment. *New England Journal of Medicine, 331*(18), 1173–1180.

Cornell, M., Majola, M., Johnson, L. F., & Dubula-Majola, V. (2021). HIV services in sub-Saharan Africa: The greatest gap is men. *The Lancet, 397*(10290), 2130–2132.

Cresswell, F. V., & Lamorde, M. (2022). Implementation of long-acting antiretroviral therapy in low-income and middle-income countries. *Current Opinion in HIV and AIDS, 17*(3), 127–134.

Cueto, M., Brown, T. M., & Fee, E. (2019). *The world health organization: A history.* Cambridge University Press, Cambridge.

Cueto, M., & Lopes, G. (2023). Braiding public health and human rights: AIDS, activism, and international agencies in Brazil, 1987–1996. *Latin American Research Review, 58*(1), 144–160.

Dabis, F., Msellati, P., Meda, N., Welffens-Ekra, C., You, B., Manigart, O., . . . Combe, P. (1999). 6-Month efficacy, tolerance, and acceptability of a short regimen of oral zido-vudine to reduce vertical transmission of HIV in breastfed children in Côte d'Ivoire and Burkina Faso: A double-blind placebo-controlled multicentre trial. *The Lancet, 353*(9155), 786–792.

DART Trial Team. (2010). Routine versus clinically driven laboratory monitoring of HIV antiretroviral therapy in Africa (DART): A randomised non-inferiority trial. *The Lancet, 375*(9709), 123–131.

Deeks, S. G., Lewin, S. R., & Havlir, D. V. (2013). The end of AIDS: HIV infection as a chronic disease. *The Lancet, 382*(9903), 1525–1533.

Dirlikov, E., Kamoga, J., Talisuna, S. A., Namusobya, J., Kasozi, D. E., Akao, J., . . . Shiraishi, R. W. (2023). Scale-up of HIV antiretroviral therapy and estimation of averted infec-tions and HIV-related deaths—Uganda, 2004–2022. *Morbidity and Mortality Weekly Report, 72*(4), 90.

Doyle, C., & Patel, P. (2008). Civil society organisations and global health initiatives: Problems of legitimacy. *Social Science & Medicine, 66*(9), 1928–1938.

Duncombe, C., Ravishankar, S., & Zuniga, J. M. (2019). Fast-track cities: Striving to end urban HIV epidemics by 2030. *Current Opinion in HIV and AIDS, 14*(6), 503–508.

Ehrenkranz, P., Grimsrud, A., Holmes, C. B., Preko, P., & Rabkin, M. (2021). Expand-ing the vision for differentiated service delivery: A call for more inclusive and truly patient-centered care for people living with HIV. *Journal of Acquired Immune Defi-ciency Syndromes (1999), 86*(2), 147.

Ehrenkranz, P., Rosen, S., Boulle, A., Eaton, J. W., Ford, N., Fox, M. P., . . . Holmes, C. B. (2021). The revolving door of HIV care: revising the service delivery cascade to achieve the UNAIDS 95-95-95 goals. *PLoS Medicine, 18*(5), e1003651.

Eisinger, R. W., Dieffenbach, C. W., & Fauci, A. S. (2019). HIV viral load and transmissi-bility of HIV infection: Undetectable equals untransmittable. *JAMA, 321*(5), 451–452.

Farrall, J., & Michaelsen, C. (2021). When the centre becomes peripheral? The UN security council's response to COVID-19. *Australian Yearbook of International Law (Forthcoming), ANU College of Law Research Paper, 21*(27), 21–78.

Feachem, R. G., & Sabot, O. J. (2006). An examination of the global fund at 5 years. *The Lancet, 368*(9534), 537–540.

Ford, N., Ball, A., Baggaley, R., Vitoria, M., Low-Beer, D., Penazzato, M., . . . Doherty, M. (2018). The WHO public health approach to HIV treatment and care: Looking back and looking ahead. *The Lancet Infectious Diseases, 18*(3), e76–e86.

Frescura, L., Godfrey-Faussett, P., Feizzadeh A, A., El-Sadr, W., Syarif, O., Ghys, P. D., . . . Group, b. o. t. t. t. W. (2022). Achieving the 95 95 95 targets for all: a pathway to ending AIDS. *Plos One, 17*(8), e0272405.

G8 Gleneagles. (2005). *G8 Gleneagles communique Africa* G8. Retrieved from http://www.g7.utoronto.ca/summit/2005gleneagles/africa.pdf

Garcia, L., & Koerner, J. (2014). Community-based responses to HIV in developed Asia: Challenges and approaches for lesbian, gay, bisexual and transgender (LGBT) people. *HIV Australia, 12*(2), 51–55.

Gilks, C., & Vitoria, M. (2006). Antiretroviral therapy for HIV infection in adults and adolescents: Recommendations for a public health approach. In *Antiretroviral therapy for HIV infection in adults and adolescents: Recommendations for a public health approach.* World Health Organization, Geneva.

Gilks, C. F. (1993). The clinical challenge of the HIV epidemic in the developing world. *The Lancet, 342*(8878), 1037–1039.

Gilks, C. F., Crowley, S., Ekpini, R., Gove, S., Perriens, J., Souteyrand, Y., . . . De Cock, K. (2006). The WHO public-health approach to antiretroviral treatment against HIV in resource-limited settings. *The Lancet, 368*(9534), 505–510.

Gilks, C. F., Floyd, K., Otieno, L. S., Adam, A. M., Bhatt, S. M., & Warrell, D. A. (1998). Some effects of the rising case load of adult HIV-related disease on a hospital in Nairobi. *Journal of Acquired Immune Deficiency Syndromes and Human Retrovirology: Official Publication of the International Retrovirology Association, 18*(3), 234–240.

Goldstein, D., Ford, N., Kisyeri, N., Munsamy, M., Nishimoto, L., Osi, K., . . . Bateganya, M. (2023). Person-centred, integrated non-communicable disease and HIV decentralized drug distribution in Eswatini and South Africa: Outcomes and challenges. *Journal of the International AIDS Society, 26*(S1), e26113. https://doi.org/10.1002/jia2.26113

Goldstein, D., Salvatore, M., Ferris, R., Phelps, B. R., & Minior, T. (2023). Integrating global HIV services with primary health care: A key step in sustainable HIV epidemic control. *The Lancet Global Health, 11*(7), e1120–e1124.

Goosby, E., Dybul, M., Fauci, A. A., Fu, J., Walsh, T., Needle, R., & Bouey, P. (2012). The United States President's emergency plan for AIDS relief: A story of partnerships and smart investments to turn the tide of the global AIDS pandemic. *Journal of Acquired Immune Deficiency Syndromes, 60*, S51–S56.

Granich, R. M., Gilks, C. F., Dye, C., De Cock, K. M., & Williams, B. G. (2009). Universal voluntary HIV testing with immediate antiretroviral therapy as a strategy for elimination of HIV transmission: A mathematical model. *The Lancet, 373*(9657), 48–57.

Green, N. C. (2022). Ending the HIV epidemic: What will happen to the HIV testing workforce? *American Journal of Public Health, 112*(4), 586–587.

Grimsrud, A., Bygrave, H., Doherty, M., Ehrenkranz, P., Ellman, T., Ferris, R., . . . Mansell, T. (2016). Reimagining HIV service delivery: The role of differentiated care from prevention to suppression. *Journal of the International AIDS Society, 19*(1), PMC5136137.

Grulich, A. E., Jin, F., Bavinton, B. R., Yeung, B., Hammoud, M. A., Amin, J., . . . Vaccher, S. (2021). Long-term protection from HIV infection with oral HIV pre-exposure prophylaxis in gay and bisexual men: Findings from the expanded and extended EPIC-NSW prospective implementation study. *The Lancet HIV, 8*(8), e486–e494.

Gruskin, S., & Tarantola, D. (2001). HIV/AIDS and human rights revisited. *Canadian HIV/AIDS Policy & Law Review, 6*(1–2), 24–29.

Haakenstad, A., Moses, M. W., Tao, T., Tsakalos, G., Zlavog, B., Kates, J., . . . Dieleman, J. L. (2019). Potential for additional government spending on HIV/AIDS in 137 low-income and middle-income countries: An economic modelling study. *The Lancet HIV, 6*(6), e382–e395.

Haberer, J. E., Mujugira, A., & Mayer, K. H. (2023). The future of HIV pre-exposure prophylaxis adherence: Reducing barriers and increasing opportunities. *The Lancet HIV, 10*(6), e404–e411.

Haines, A., & Cassels, A. (2004). Can the millennium development goals be attained? *BMJ, 329*(7462), 394–397.

Hankins, C. A., & de Zalduondo, B. O. (2010). Combination prevention: A deeper understanding of effective HIV prevention. *AIDS, 24*, S70–S80.

Hayes, R. J., Donnell, D., Floyd, S., Mandla, N., Bwalya, J., Sabapathy, K., . . . Eshleman, S. H. (2019). Effect of universal testing and treatment on HIV incidence— HPTN 071 (PopART). *New England Journal of Medicine, 381*(3), 207–218.

Honermann, B., Bass, E., & Millett, G. (2023). Failing to learn the lessons: The US response on global health security ignores 20 years of PEPFAR. *Journal of the International AIDS Society, 26*(6), PMC10233363.

Insight Start Study Group. (2015). Initiation of antiretroviral therapy in early asymptomatic HIV infection. *New England Journal of Medicine, 373*(9), 795–807.

INSIGHT Strategic Timing of AntiRetroviral Treatment Study Group. (2023). Long-Term Benefits from Early Antiretroviral Therapy Initiation in HIV Infection. *NEJM Evidence, 2*(3), EVIDoa2200302.

Izudi, J., Kiragga, A. N., Okoboi, S., Bajunirwe, F., & Castelnuovo, B. (2022). Adaptations to HIV services delivery amidst the COVID-19 pandemic restrictions in Kampala, Uganda: A qualitative study. *PLOS Global Public Health, 2*(8), e0000908.

Joint UNAIDS Programme on HIV/AIDS (UNAIDS). (2023). *The path that ends AIDS: UNAIDS Global AIDS update 2023.* Geneva

Joint United Nations Programme on AIDS (UNAIDS). (2007). *Practical guidelines for intensifying HIV prevention: Towards universal access.* (9291736139). World Health Organization, Geneva.

Joint United Nations Programme on HIV/AIDS (UNAIDS). (2006). *International Guidelines on HIV/AIDS and Human Rights.*

Joint United Nations Programme on HIV/AIDS (UNAIDS). (2008). *2008 report on the global AIDS epidemic.* World Health Organization, Geneva.

Joint United Nations Programme on HIV/AIDS (UNAIDS). (2010). *Getting to zero: 2011–2015 strategy.* World Health Organization, Geneva.

Joint United Nations Programme on HIV/AIDS (UNAIDS). (2015). *Understanding fast-track: Accelerating action to end the AIDS epidemic by 2030.*

Joint United Nations Programme on HIV/AIDS (UNAIDS). (2022). *In danger: UNAIDS global AIDS update 2022.* (9210019792). UN

Kaleeba, N., & Ray, S. (2003). We miss you all. Noerine Kaleeba: AIDS in the family. *Reproductive Health Matters, 11*(22), 187–191.

Kassanjee, R., Davies, M. A., Ngwenya, O., Osei-Yeboah, R., Jacobs, T., Morden, E., . . . Taljaard, J. (2023). COVID-19 among adults living with HIV: Correlates of mortality among public sector healthcare users in Western Cape, South Africa. *Journal of the International AIDS Society, 26*(6), e26104.

Kates, J., Wexler, A., & Lief, E. (2014). *Financing the response to HIV in low and middle-income countries.* Kaiser Family Foundation, Menlo Park, CA.

Kayal, P. M. (2018). *Bearing witness: Gay men's health crisis and the politics of AIDS.* Routledge.

Kim, J. Y., & Ammann, A. (2004). Is the "3 by 5" initiative the best approach to tackling the HIV pandemic? *PLoS Medicine, 1*(2), e37.

Kurth, A. E., Celum, C., Baeten, J. M., Vermund, S. H., & Wasserheit, J. N. (2011). Combination HIV prevention: Significance, challenges, and opportunities. *Current HIV/ AIDS Reports, 8*, 62–72.

Lallemant, M., Jourdain, G., Le Coeur, S., Kim, S., Koetsawang, S., Comeau, A. M., . . . Vithayasai, V. (2000). A trial of shortened zidovudine regimens to prevent mother-to-child transmission of human immunodeficiency virus type 1. *New England Journal of Medicine*, *343*(14), 982–991.

Lancet. (2005). Maintaining anti-AIDS commitment post "3 by 5". *The Lancet*, *366*(9500), 1828.

Le Blanc, D. (2015). Towards integration at last? The sustainable development goals as a network of targets. *Sustainable Development*, *23*(3), 176–187.

Lee, J.-W. (2003). Global health improvement and WHO: Shaping the future. *The Lancet*, *362*(9401), 2083–2088.

Liegeon, G., & Ghosn, J. (2022). Long-acting injectable cabotegravir for PrEP: A game-changer in HIV prevention? *HIV Medicine*, *24*(6), 653–663.

Long, L., Kuchukhidze, S., Pascoe, S., Nichols, B. E., Fox, M. P., Cele, R., . . . Rosen, S. (2020). Retention in care and viral suppression in differentiated service delivery models for HIV treatment delivery in sub-Saharan Africa: A rapid systematic review. *Journal of the International AIDS Society*, *23*(11), e25640.

Manoto, S. L., Lugongolo, M., Govender, U., & Mthunzi-Kufa, P. (2018). Point of care diagnostics for HIV in resource limited settings: An overview. *Medicina*, *54*(1), 3.

McGuire, M., de Waal, A., Karellis, A., Janssen, R., Engel, N., Sampath, R., . . . Pai, N. P. (2021). HIV self-testing with digital supports as the new paradigm: A systematic review of global evidence (2010–2021). *EClinicalMedicine*, *39*, 101059.

Merianos, A., & Peiris, M. (2005). International health regulations (2005). *The Lancet*, *366*(9493), 1249–1251.

Mitchell, V. S., Philipose, N. M., & Sanford, J. P. (1993). *The children's vaccine initiative: Achieving the vision*. National Academies Press, Washington, DC.

Molina, J.-M., Charreau, I., Spire, B., Cotte, L., Chas, J., Capitant, C., . . . Pasquet, A. (2017). Efficacy, safety, and effect on sexual behaviour of on-demand pre-exposure prophylaxis for HIV in men who have sex with men: An observational cohort study. *The Lancet HIV*, *4*(9), e402–e410.

Morolake, O., Stephens, D., & Welbourn, A. (2009). Greater involvement of people living with HIV in health care. *Journal of the International AIDS Society*, *12*, 1–7.

Musaazi, J., Sekaggya-Wiltshire, C., Okoboi, S., Zawedde-Muyanja, S., Senkoro, M., Kalema, N., . . . Castelnuovo, B. (2023). Increased uptake of tuberculosis preventive therapy (TPT) among people living with HIV following the 100-days accelerated campaign: A retrospective review of routinely collected data at six urban public health facilities in Uganda. *Plos One*, *18*(2), e0268935.

Musekiwa, A., Fernando, N. B., & Abariga, S. A. (2020). Effectiveness of vaginal microbicides in preventing HIV transmission. *Tropical Medicine & International Health*, *25*(7), 790–802.

Nachega, J. B., Adetokunboh, O., Uthman, O. A., Knowlton, A. W., Altice, F. L., Schechter, M., . . . Chang, L. W. (2016). Community-based interventions to improve and sustain antiretroviral therapy adherence, retention in HIV care and clinical outcomes in low-and middle-income countries for achieving the UNAIDS 90-90-90 targets. *Current HIV/AIDS Reports*, *13*, 241–255.

Nachega, J. B., Scarsi, K. K., Gandhi, M., Scott, R. K., Mofenson, L. M., Archary, M., . . . Wilson, L. (2023). Long-acting antiretrovirals and HIV treatment adherence. *The Lancet HIV*, *10*(5), e332–e342.

Ngari, M. M., Rashid, M. A., Sanga, D., Mathenge, H., Agoro, O., Mberia, J. K., . . . Abdullahi, O. A. (2023). Burden of HIV and treatment outcomes among TB patients in rural Kenya: A 9-year longitudinal study. *BMC Infectious Diseases, 23*(1), 1–11.

Paton, N. I., Musaazi, J., Kityo, C., Walimbwa, S., Hoppe, A., Balyegisawa, A., . . . Ategeka, G. (2021). Dolutegravir or darunavir in combination with zidovudine or tenofovir to treat HIV. *New England Journal of Medicine, 385*(4), 330–341.

Pepin, J. (2011). *The Origins of AIDS.* Cambridge University Press, Cambridge.

Quinn, T., Wawer, M., Sewankambo, N., Serwadda, D., Li, C., & Wabwire-Mangen, F. (2000). Viral load and heterosexual transmission of HIV type 1. Rakai Project Study Group. *New England Journal of Medicine, 342*(13), 921–929.

Rodi, P., Obermeyer, W., Pablos-Mendez, A., Gori, A., & Raviglione, M. C. (2022). Political rationale, aims, and outcomes of health-related high-level meetings and special sessions at the UN General Assembly: A policy research observational study. *PLoS Medicine, 19*(1), e1003873.

Sachs, J. D. (2012). From millennium development goals to sustainable development goals. *The Lancet, 379*(9832), 2206–2211.

Santosa, A., Wall, S., Fottrell, E., Högberg, U., & Byass, P. (2014). The development and experience of epidemiological transition theory over four decades: A systematic review. *Global Health Action, 7*(1), 23574.

Schulman, S. (2021). *Let the record show: A political history of ACT UP New York, 1987–1993.* Farrar, Straus and Giroux, New York.

Schwartländer, B., Stover, J., Walker, N., Bollinger, L., Gutierrez, J. P., McGreevey, W., . . . Watts, C. (2001). Resource needs for HIV/AIDS. *Science, 292*(5526), 2434–2436.

Sgaier, S. K., Claeson, M., Gilks, C., Ramesh, B. M., Ghys, P. D., Wadhwani, A., . . . Chandramouli, K. (2012). Knowing your HIV/AIDS epidemic and tailoring an effective response: How did India do it? *Sexually Transmitted Infections, 88*(4), 240–249.

Siedner, M. J., Moosa, M.-Y. S., McCluskey, S., Gilbert, R. F., Pillay, S., Aturinda, I., . . . Masette, G. (2021). Resistance testing for management of HIV virologic failure in sub-Saharan Africa: An unblinded randomized controlled trial. *Annals of Internal Medicine, 174*(12), 1683–1692.

Smith, J. H., & Whiteside, A. (2010). The history of AIDS exceptionalism. *Journal of the International AIDS Society, 13*(1), 1–8.

Strategies for Management of Antiretroviral Therapy Study Group. (2008). Inferior clinical outcome of the CD4+ cell count–guided antiretroviral treatment interruption strategy in the SMART study: Role of CD4+ cell counts and HIV RNA levels during follow-up. *The Journal of Infectious Diseases, 197*(8), 1145–1155.

Suthar, A. B., Vitoria, M. A., Nagata, J. M., Anglaret, X., Mbori-Ngacha, D., Sued, O., . . . Doherty, M. C. (2015). Co-trimoxazole prophylaxis in adults, including pregnant women, with HIV: A systematic review and meta-analysis. *The Lancet HIV, 2*(4), e137–e150.

Swindells, S., Andrade-Villanueva, J.-F., Richmond, G. J., Rizzardini, G., Baumgarten, A., Masiá, M., . . . Smith, G. (2020). Long-acting cabotegravir and rilpivirine for maintenance of HIV-1 suppression. *New England Journal of Medicine, 382*(12), 1112–1123.

Szijarto, S. (2023). Activism and Authority: ACT UP and TAC as Successful Arbiters of HIV Treatment Policy Change. *Aletheia, 3*(1). https://doi.org/10.15173/a.v3i1.3397

Trickey, A., Sabin, C. A., Burkholder, G., Crane, H., Monforte, A. d. A., Egger, M., . . . Jarrin, I. (2023). Life expectancy after 2015 of adults with HIV on long-term antiretroviral therapy in Europe and North America: A collaborative analysis of cohort studies. *The Lancet HIV, 10*(5), e295–e307.

Tynkkynen, L.-K., Keskimäki, I., & Lehto, J. (2013). Purchaser–provider splits in health care—The case of Finland. *Health Policy, 111*(3), 221–225.

UNAIDS & WHO. (2004). *UNAIDS/WHO Policy Statement on HIV Testing.* Geneva.

Ungurean, C. (2005). *Millennium Development Goals.*

United Nations (UN). (2000a). RES. 55/2. United Nations Millennium Declaration. *Fifty fifth United Nations General Assembly, New York, 18 September 2000.* Retrieved from www.un.org/en/development/desa/population/migration/generalassembly/docs/globalcompact/A_RES_55_2.pdf

United Nations (UN). (2000b). Resolution 1308 (2000) Adopted by the Security Council at its 4172nd Meeting, on 17 July 2000. In: Security Council, UN New York.

United Nations (UN). (2001). *Declaration of Commitment on HIV/AIDS: Resolution adopted by the UNSC 17 July 2000.* Retrieved from https://digitallibrary.un.org/record/443771

United Nations (UN). (2006). *Resolution adopted by the General Assembly: 60/262. Political Declaration on HIV/AIDS.* A/RES/60/262.

United Nations (UN). (2011). *Political declaration on HIV/AIDS: Intensifying our efforts to eliminate HIV/AIDS.* UNAIDS Geneva.

United Nations (UN). (2021). *Political declaration on HIV and AIDS: Ending inequalities and getting on track to end AIDS by 2030.*

Van Lerberghe, W. (2008). *The world health report 2008: Primary health care: Now more than ever.* World Health Organization, Geneva.

Waife, N., Witter, S., & Jones, S. (2019). Evaluation of DFID's Approach to Making Country Health Systems Stronger (MCHSS) Literature Review Report.

Waitzkin, H. (2003). Report of the WHO Commission on Macroeconomics and Health: A summary and critique. *The Lancet, 361*(9356), 523–526.

Wilson, D., & Halperin, D. T. (2008). "Know your epidemic, know your response": A useful approach, if we get it right. *The Lancet, 372*(9637), 423–426.

World Health Organization (WHO). (1986). Acquired immunodeficiency syndrome (AIDS): WHO/CDC case definition for AIDS. *Weekly Epidemiological Record= Relevé épidémiologique hebdomadaire, 61*(10), 69–74.

World Health Organization (WHO). (2002a). *Implications of the Doha Declaration on the TRIPS Agreement and public health.* Retrieved from https://apps.who.int/iris/bitstream/handle/10665/67345/WHO_EDM_PAR_2002.3.pdf

World Health Organization (WHO). (2002b). *Scaling up antiretroviral therapy in resource-limited settings: Guidelines for a public health approach: Executive summary* (9241545674). Retrieved from https://apps.who.int/iris/handle/10665/42514

World Health Organization (WHO). (2003a). *A public health approach to antiretroviral treatment: Overcoming constraints.* World Health Organization, Geneva.

World Health Organization (WHO). (2003b). *Treating 3 million by 2005: Making it happen: The WHO strategy: The WHO and UNAIDS global initiative to provide antiretroviral therapy to 3 million people with HIV/AIDS in developing countries by the end of 2005/Treat 3 Million by 2005 Initiative.* Retrieved from https://data.unaids.org/publications/external-documents/who_3by5-strategy_en.pdf

World Health Organization (WHO). (2004a). *Chronic HIV care with ARV therapy, integrated management of adolescent and adult illness, interim guidelines for first-level facility health workers.*

World Health Organization (WHO). (2004b). *The World health report: 2004: Changing history*. World Health Organization, Geneva.

World Health Organization (WHO). (2006a). Antiretroviral drugs for treating pregnant women and preventing HIV infection in infants in resource-limited settings: Towards universal access: Recommendations for a public health approach.

World Health Organization (WHO). (2006b). *Guidelines on co-trimoxazole prophylaxis for HIV-related infections among children, adolescents and adults in resource-limited settings: Recommendations for a public health approach.* (9241594705).

World Health Organization (WHO). (2006c). *Management of HIV infection and antiretroviral therapy in infants and children: A clinical manual.* (9290222840). WHO Regional Office for South-East Asia

World Health Organization (WHO). (2006d). *Progress on global access to HIV antiretroviral therapy: A report on "3 by 5" and beyond, March 2006.* (9241594136).

World Health Organization (WHO). (2007a). Guidance on provider-initiated HIV testing and counselling in health facilities.

World Health Organization (WHO). (2007b). *People-centred health care: A policy framework* (9789290613176).

World Health Organization (WHO). (2007c). *Task shifting: Rational redistribution of tasks among health workforce teams: Global recommendations and guidelines.* (9241596317).

World Health Organization (WHO). (2007d). *WHO case definitions of HIV for surveillance and revised clinical staging and immunological classification of HIV-related disease in adults and children*. World Health Organization, Geneva.

World Health Organization (WHO). (2013). *Consolidated guidelines on general HIV care and the use of antiretroviral drugs for treating and preventing HIV infection: Recommendations for a public health approach*. World Health Organization, Geneva, 269.

World Health Organization (WHO). (2014a). *Access to antiretroviral drugs in low-and middle-income countries: Technical report July 2014.* (9241507543).

World Health Organization (WHO). (2014b). *WHO handbook for guideline development*. World Health Organization, Geneva.

World Health Organization (WHO). (2015a). Consolidated guidelines on HIV testing services: 5Cs: Consent, confidentiality, counselling, correct results and connection 2015.

World Health Organization (WHO). (2015b). *Policy brief: Pre-exposure prophylaxis (PrEP): WHO expands recommendation on oral pre-exposure prophylaxis of HIV infection (PrEP)*. World Health Organization, Geneva.

World Health Organization (WHO). (2015c). *World health statistics 2015*. World Health Organization, Geneva.

World Health Organization (WHO). (2017a). *Guidelines for managing advanced HIV disease and rapid initiation of antiretroviral therapy, July 2017.* (9241550066).

World Health Organization (WHO). (2017b). *World health statistics 2017: Monitoring health for the SDGs.*

World Health Organization (WHO). (2018). *HIV self-testing strategic framework: A guide for planning, introducing and scaling up*. World Health Organization, Geneva.

World Health Organization (WHO). (2019). *WHO Medicines, Vaccines and Pharmaceuticals (MVP) 2018 annual report: Promoting access to safe, effective, quality and affordable essential medical products for all*. World Health Organization, Geneva.

World Health Organization (WHO). (2020). *Consolidated HIV strategic information guidelines: Driving impact through programme monitoring and management.*

World Health Organization (WHO). (2021). *Consolidated guidelines on HIV prevention, testing, treatment, service delivery and monitoring: Recommendations for a public health approach.* World Health Organization, Geneva.

World Health Organization (WHO). (2023a). *Integrating the prevention and control of noncommunicable diseases in HIV.*

World Health Organization (WHO). (2023b). *Integration of noncommunicable diseases into HIV service packages: Technical brief.*

World Health Organization (WHO). (2023c). *Primary health care and HIV: Convergent actions: Policy considerations for decision-makers.*

Zarocostas, J. (2023). With the COVID-19 PHEIC over, what next? *The Lancet, 401*(10389), 1642–1643.

Section 2

Allen, L. N. (2017). Financing national non-communicable disease responses. *Global Health Action, 10*(1), 1326687.

Assefa, Y., & Gilks, C. F. (2020). Ending the epidemic of HIV/AIDS by 2030: Will there be an endgame to HIV, or an endemic HIV requiring an integrated health systems response in many countries? *International Journal of Infectious Diseases, 100*, 273–277.

Banatvala, N., Akselrod, S., Bovet, P., & Mendis, S. (2023). The WHO global action plan for the prevention and control of NCDs 2013–2030. In *Noncommunicable diseases* (pp. 234–239). Routledge.

Beaglehole, R., Bonita, R., Alleyne, G., Horton, R., Li, L., Lincoln, P., . . . Nishtar, S. (2011). UN high-level meeting on non-communicable diseases: Addressing four questions. *The Lancet, 378*(9789), 449–455.

Beaglehole, R., Bonita, R., Horton, R., Adams, C., Alleyne, G., Asaria, P., . . . Casswell, S. (2011). Priority actions for the non-communicable disease crisis. *The Lancet, 377*(9775), 1438–1447.

Beaglehole, R., Ebrahim, S., Reddy, S., Voûte, J., & Leeder, S. (2007). Prevention of chronic diseases: A call to action. *The Lancet, 370*(9605), 2152–2157.

Beaglehole, R., & Horton, R. (2010). Chronic diseases: Global action must match global evidence. *The Lancet, 376*(9753), 1619–1621.

Bennett, J. E., Stevens, G. A., Mathers, C. D., Bonita, R., Rehm, J., Kruk, M. E., . . . Chalkidou, K. (2018). NCD Countdown 2030: Worldwide trends in non-communicable disease mortality and progress towards Sustainable Development Goal target 3.4. *The Lancet, 392*(10152), 1072–1088.

Bloom, D. E., Khoury, A., & Subbaraman, R. (2018). The promise and peril of universal health care. *Science, 361*(6404), eaat9644.

Bonita, R., Winkelmann, R., Douglas, K. A., & de Courten, M. (2003). The WHO Stepwise approach to surveillance (STEPS) of non-communicable disease risk factors. In *Global behavioral risk factor surveillance* (pp. 9–22). Springer.

Bousquet, J., Kiley, J., Bateman, E., Viegi, G., Cruz, A., Khaltaev, N., . . . Billo, N. (2010). Prioritised research agenda for prevention and control of chronic respiratory diseases. *European Respiratory Journal, 36*(5), 995–1001.

Bray, G. A. (2006). Obesity: The disease. *Journal of medicinal chemistry*, *49*(14), 4001–4007.

Brownell, K. D., Farley, T., Willett, W. C., Popkin, B. M., Chaloupka, F. J., Thompson, J. W., & Ludwig, D. S. (2009). The public health and economic benefits of taxing sugar-sweetened beverages. *The New England Journal of Medicine*, *361*(16), 1599.

Bullen, C., McCormack, J., Calder, A., Parag, V., Subramaniam, K., Majumdar, A., . . . Goodyear-Smith, F. (2021). The impact of COVID-19 on the care of people living with noncommunicable diseases in low-and middle-income countries: An online survey of physicians and pharmacists in nine countries. *Primary Health Care Research & Development*, *22*, e30.

Cecchini, M., Sassi, F., Lauer, J. A., Lee, Y. Y., Guajardo-Barron, V., & Chisholm, D. (2010). Tackling of unhealthy diets, physical inactivity, and obesity: Health effects and cost-effectiveness. *The Lancet*, *376*(9754), 1775–1784.

Das, J., Chowdhury, A., Hussam, R., & Banerjee, A. V. (2016). The impact of training informal health care providers in India: A randomized controlled trial. *Science*, *354*(6308), aaf7384.

Dieleman, J. L., Schneider, M. T., Haakenstad, A., Singh, L., Sadat, N., Birger, M., . . . Chapin, A. (2016). Development assistance for health: Past trends, associations, and the future of international financial flows for health. *The Lancet*, *387*(10037), 2536–2544.

Ezzati, M., & Riboli, E. (2012). Can noncommunicable diseases be prevented? Lessons from studies of populations and individuals. *Science*, *337*(6101), 1482–1487.

Frenk, J. (2010). The global health system: Strengthening national health systems as the next step for global progress. *PLoS Medicine*, *7*(1), e1000089.

Gaziano, T. A., Galea, G., & Reddy, K. S. (2007). Scaling up interventions for chronic disease prevention: The evidence. *The Lancet*, *370*(9603), 1939–1946.

Geneau, R., Stuckler, D., Stachenko, S., McKee, M., Ebrahim, S., Basu, S., . . . Alwan, A. (2010). Raising the priority of preventing chronic diseases: A political process. *The Lancet*, *376*(9753), 1689–1698.

Gilks, C. F., Crowley, S., Ekpini, R., Gove, S., Perriens, J., Souteyrand, Y., . . . De Cock, K. (2006). The WHO public-health approach to antiretroviral treatment against HIV in resource-limited settings. *The Lancet*, *368*(9534), 505–510.

Hanson, K., Brikci, N., Erlangga, D., Alebachew, A., De Allegri, M., Balabanova, D., . . . Hipgrave, D. (2022). The Lancet Global Health Commission on financing primary health care: Putting people at the centre. *The Lancet Global Health*, *10*(5), e715–e772.

Harrison, J. E., Weber, S., Jakob, R., & Chute, C. G. (2021). ICD-11: An international classification of diseases for the twenty-first century. *BMC Medical Informatics and Decision Making*, *21*(6), 1–10.

He, J., Ouyang, N., Guo, X., Sun, G., Li, Z., Mu, J., . . . Ren, G. (2023). Effectiveness of a non-physician community health-care provider-led intensive blood pressure intervention versus usual care on cardiovascular disease (CRHCP): An open-label, blinded-endpoint, cluster-randomised trial. *The Lancet*, *401*(10380), 928–938.

Horton, R. (2007). Chronic diseases: The case for urgent global action. *The Lancet*, *370*(9603), 1881–1882.

Jailobaeva, K., Falconer, J., Loffreda, G., Arakelyan, S., Witter, S., & Ager, A. (2021). An analysis of policy and funding priorities of global actors regarding noncommunicable disease in low-and middle-income countries. *Globalization and Health*, *17*(1), 1–15.

Jamison, D. T., Alwan, A., Mock, C. N., Nugent, R., Watkins, D., Adeyi, O., . . . Bhutta, Z. (2018). Universal health coverage and intersectoral action for health: Key messages from Disease Control Priorities. *The Lancet*, *391*(10125), 1108–1120.

Jamison, D. T., & Mosley, W. H. (1991). Disease control priorities in developing countries: Health policy responses to epidemiological change. *American Journal of Public Health*, *81*(1), 15–22.

Jamison, D. T., Summers, L. H., Alleyne, G., Arrow, K. J., Berkley, S., Binagwaho, A., . . . Frenk, J. (2013). Global health 2035: A world converging within a generation. *The Lancet*, *382*(9908), 1898–1955.

Joseph, P., Leong, D., McKee, M., Anand, S. S., Schwalm, J.-D., Teo, K., . . . Yusuf, S. (2017). Reducing the global burden of cardiovascular disease, part 1: The epidemiology and risk factors. *Circulation Research*, *121*(6), 677–694.

Joseph, P., Roshandel, G., Gao, P., Pais, P., Lonn, E., Xavier, D., . . . Sliwa, K. (2021). Fixed-dose combination therapies with and without aspirin for primary prevention of cardiovascular disease: An individual participant data meta-analysis. *The Lancet*, *398*(10306), 1133–1146.

Kamenov, K., Mills, J.-A., Chatterji, S., & Cieza, A. (2019). Needs and unmet needs for rehabilitation services: A scoping review. *Disability and rehabilitation*, *41*(10), 1227–1237.

Kankeu, H. T., Saksena, P., Xu, K., & Evans, D. B. (2013). The financial burden from non-communicable diseases in low-and middle-income countries: A literature review. *Health Research Policy and Systems*, *11*(1), 1–12.

Karppanen, H., & Mervaala, E. (2006). Sodium intake and hypertension. *Progress in Cardiovascular Diseases*, *49*(2), 59–75.

Kokkinos, P., Sheriff, H., & Kheirbek, R. (2011). Physical inactivity and mortality risk. *Cardiology Research and Practice*, *2011*, 924945.

L. Allen, S. Wigley, H. Holmer, & Barlow., P. (2023). Non-communicable disease policy implementation from 2014 to 2021: A repeated cross-sectional analysis of global policy data for 194 countries. *The Lancet Global Health*, *11*(4), e525–e533.

Lassi, Z. S., Salam, R. A., Das, J. K., & Bhutta, Z. A. (2014). Essential interventions for maternal, newborn and child health: Background and methodology. *Reproductive Health*, *11*(1), 1–7.

Laxminarayan, R., Mills, A. J., Breman, J. G., Measham, A. R., Alleyne, G., Claeson, M., . . . Shahid-Salles, S. (2006). Advancement of global health: Key messages from the Disease Control Priorities Project. *The Lancet*, *367*(9517), 1193–1208.

Linou, N., Beagley, J., Huikuri, S., & Renshaw, N. (2018). *Air pollution moves up the global health agenda*, Vol. 363. British Medical Journal Publishing Group.

Lozano, R., Fullman, N., Abate, D., Abay, S. M., Abbafati, C., Abbasi, N., . . . Abdelalim, A. (2018). Measuring progress from 1990 to 2017 and projecting attainment to 2030 of the health-related Sustainable Development Goals for 195 countries and territories: A systematic analysis for the Global Burden of Disease Study 2017. *The Lancet*, *392*(10159), 2091–2138.

Marmot, M. G., Stansfeld, S., Patel, C., North, F., Head, J., White, I., . . . Smith, G. D. (1991). Health inequalities among British civil servants: The Whitehall II study. *The Lancet*, *337*(8754), 1387–1393.

Michas, G., Micha, R., & Zampelas, A. (2014). Dietary fats and cardiovascular disease: Putting together the pieces of a complicated puzzle. *Atherosclerosis*, *234*(2), 320–328.

Mills, A. (2014). Health care systems in low-and middle-income countries. *New England Journal of Medicine, 370*(6), 552–557.

Mock, C. N., Donkor, P., Gawande, A., Jamison, D. T., Kruk, M. E., & Debas, H. T. (2015). Essential surgery: Key messages from Disease Control Priorities. *The Lancet, 385*(9983), 2209–2219.

Murray, C. J., & Lopez, A. D. (1996). *The global burden of disease: A comprehensive assessment of mortality and disability from diseases, injuries, and risk factors in 1990 and projected to 2020: Summary.* World Health Organization, Geneva.

Nugent, R. (2016). A chronology of global assistance funding for NCD. *Global Heart, 11*(4), 371–374.

Omran, A. R. (1998). The epidemiologic transition theory revisited thirty years later. *World Health Statistics Quarterly, 53*(2, 3, 4), 99–119.

Patel, V., Saxena, S., Lund, C., Thornicroft, G., Baingana, F., Bolton, P., . . . Eaton, J. (2018). The Lancet Commission on global mental health and sustainable development. *The Lancet, 392*(10157), 1553–1598.

Rodgers, A., & Smith, R. (2023). *The polypill and medicines access: Two decades and counting,* Vol. 382. British Medical Journal Publishing Group.

Rodi, P., Obermeyer, W., Pablos-Mendez, A., Gori, A., & Raviglione, M. C. (2022). Political rationale, aims, and outcomes of health-related high-level meetings and special sessions at the UN General Assembly: A policy research observational study. *PLoS Medicine, 19*(1), e1003873.

Roglic, G. (2016). WHO Global report on diabetes: A summary. *International Journal of Noncommunicable Diseases, 1*(1), 3–8.

Rumbold, B., Baker, R., Ferraz, O., Hawkes, S., Krubiner, C., Littlejohns, P., . . . Venkatapuram, S. (2017). Universal health coverage, priority setting, and the human right to health. *The Lancet, 390*(10095), 712–714.

Samb, B., Desai, N., Nishtar, S., Mendis, S., Bekedam, H., Wright, A., . . . Patel, K. (2010). Prevention and management of chronic disease: A litmus test for health-systems strengthening in low-income and middle-income countries. *The Lancet, 376*(9754), 1785–1797.

Santosa, A., Wall, S., Fottrell, E., Högberg, U., & Byass, P. (2014). The development and experience of epidemiological transition theory over four decades: A systematic review. *Global Health Action, 7*(1), 23574.

Strong, K., Mathers, C., Leeder, S., & Beaglehole, R. (2005). Preventing chronic diseases: How many lives can we save? *The Lancet, 366*(9496), 1578–1582.

Swinburn, B. A., Kraak, V. I., Allender, S., Atkins, V. J., Baker, P. I., Bogard, J. R., . . . Devarajan, R. (2019). The global syndemic of obesity, undernutrition, and climate change: The Lancet Commission report. *The Lancet, 393*(10173), 791–846.

Thakur, J. S., Nangia, R., & Singh, S. (2021). Progress and challenges in achieving non-communicable diseases targets for the sustainable development goals. *FASEB BioAdvances, 3*(8), 563.

United Nations (UN). (2011). *Political declaration of the high-level meeting of the general assembly on the prevention and control of non-communicable diseases.*

United Nations (UN). (2014). United Nations General Assembly: 68th Session Agenda Item 118 Outcome Document of the High-Level Meeting of the General Assembly on the Comprehensive Review and Assessment of the Progress Achieved in the Prevention and Control of Non-Communicable Diseases. United Nations New York, NY.

United Nations (UN). (2015). *Transforming our world: The 2030 Agenda for Sustainable Development.*

United Nations (UN). (2018). *Political declaration of the third high-level meeting of the General Assembly on the prevention and control of non-communicable diseases.*

Vos, T., Lim, S. S., Abbafati, C., Abbas, K. M., Abbasi, M., Abbasifard, M., . . . Abdelalim, A. (2020). Global burden of 369 diseases and injuries in 204 countries and territories, 1990–2019: A systematic analysis for the Global Burden of Disease Study 2019. *The Lancet, 396*(10258), 1204–1222.

Watkins, D. A., Msemburi, W. T., Pickersgill, S. J., Kawakatsu, Y., Gheorghe, A., Dain, K., . . . Tolla, M. T. (2022). NCD Countdown 2030: Efficient pathways and strategic investments to accelerate progress towards the Sustainable Development Goal target 3.4 in low-income and middle-income countries. *The Lancet, 399*(10331), 1266–1278.

WHO Commission on Social Determinants of Health. (2008). *Closing the gap in a generation: Health equity through action on the social determinants of health: Commission on Social Determinants of Health final report.* World Health Organization, Geneva.

Wild, C. P. (2012). The role of cancer research in noncommunicable disease control. *Journal of the National Cancer Institute, 104*(14), 1051–1058.

World Health Organization (WHO). (2002). *The world health report 2002: Reducing risks, promoting healthy life.* World Health Organization, Geneva.

World Health Organization (WHO). (2005a). *Preventing chronic diseases: A vital investment.* (9241563001). World Health Organization, Geneva.

World Health Organization (WHO). (2005b). *WHO STEPS surveillance manual: The WHO STEPwise approach to chronic disease risk factor surveillance.* World Health Organization, Geneva.

World Health Organization (WHO). (2010). *Global strategy to reduce the harmful use of alcohol.* World Health Organization, Geneva.

World Health Organization (WHO). (2013). *Global action plan for the prevention and control of noncommunicable diseases 2013–2020.* World Health Organization, Geneva.

World Health Organization (WHO). (2017). *Tackling NCDs: 'best buys' and other recommended interventions for the prevention and control of noncommunicable diseases.*

World Health Organization (WHO). (2018a). *Antimicrobial resistance and primary health care.* World Health Organization, Geneva.

World Health Organization (WHO). (2018b). *Technical package for cardiovascular disease management in primary health care: Implementation guide.*

World Health Organization (WHO). (2018c). *Time to deliver: Report of the WHO independent high-level commission on noncommunicable diseases.* World Health Organization, Geneva.

World Health Organization (WHO). (2019a). *General meeting of the WHO global coordination mechanism on the prevention and control of noncommunicable diseases: Meeting report: International Conference Centre, Geneva, Switzerland, 5–6 November 2018.*

World Health Organization (WHO). (2019b). *It's Time to Walk the Talk: WHO Independent High-Level Commission on Noncommunicable Diseases Final Report.* WHO, Geneva.

World Health Organization (WHO). (2020). *WHO package of essential noncommunicable (PEN) disease interventions for primary health care.* (9240009221).

World Health Organization (WHO). (2021a). *Comprehensive mental health action plan 2013–2030.*

World Health Organization (WHO). (2021b). *Nothing for us, without us: Opportunities for meaningful engagement of people living with NCDs: Meeting report.*

World Health Organization (WHO). (2022a). *Noncommunicable diseases. Fact sheet 13 April 2021.*

World Health Organization (WHO). (2022b). *Noncommunicable diseases: Progress monitor 2022.* (924004776X).

World Health Organization (WHO). (2023a). *Advancing the global agenda on prevention and control of noncommunicable diseases 2000 to 2020: Looking forwards to 2030.* (9240072691).

World Health Organization (WHO). (2023b). *Building an NCD-ready workforce: Technical meeting report, Geneva, Switzerland, 3–4 June 2021.* World Health Organization, Geneva.

World Health Organization (WHO). (2023c). *Global report on neglected tropical diseases 2023: Executive summary* (9240069011).

World Health Organization (WHO). (2023d). *Integrating the prevention and control of noncommunicable diseases in HIV.*

World Health Organization (WHO). (2023e). *WHO report on the global tobacco epidemic, 2023: Protect people from tobacco smoke.*

Zhu, J. Z., Manne-Goehler, J., Agarwal, A., Bahendeka, S. K., Damasceno, A., Marcus, M. E., . . . Flood, D. (2023). Medication use for cardiovascular disease prevention in 40 low-and middle-income countries. *Journal of the American College of Cardiology, 81*(6), 620–622.

Section 3

Abiiro, G. A., Mbera, G. B., & De Allegri, M. (2014). Gaps in universal health coverage in Malawi: A qualitative study in rural communities. *BMC Health Services Research, 14*, 1–10.

Abimbola, S., Baatiema, L., & Bigdeli, M. (2019). The impacts of decentralization on health system equity, efficiency and resilience: A realist synthesis of the evidence. *Health Policy and Planning, 34*(8), 605–617.

Adebisi, Y. A., Nwogu, I. B., Alaran, A. J., Badmos, A. O., Bamgboye, A. O., Rufai, B. O., . . . Abdalla, S. F. (2022). Revisiting the issue of access to medicines in Africa: Challenges and recommendations. *Public Health Challenges, 1*(2), e9.

Afriyie, D. O., Hooley, B., Mhalu, G., Tediosi, F., & Mtenga, S. M. (2021). Governance factors that affect the implementation of health financing reforms in Tanzania: An exploratory study of stakeholders' perspectives. *BMJ Global Health, 6*(8), e005964.

Agustina, R., Dartanto, T., Sitompul, R., Susiloretni, K. A., Achadi, E. L., Taher, A., . . . Shankar, A. H. (2019). Universal health coverage in Indonesia: Concept, progress, and challenges. *The Lancet, 393*(10166), 75–102.

Agyepong, I., Spicer, N., Ooms, G., Jahn, A., Bärnighausen, T., Beiersmann, C., . . . Hennig, L. (2023). Lancet Commission on synergies between universal health coverage, health security, and health promotion. *The Lancet, 401*(10392), 1964–2012.

Agyepong, I. A., Abankwah, D. N. Y., Abroso, A., Chun, C., Dodoo, J. N. O., Lee, S., . . . Oh, J. (2016). The "Universal" in UHC and Ghana's National Health Insurance Scheme: Policy and implementation challenges and dilemmas of a lower middle income country. *BMC Health Services Research, 16*(1), 1–14.

Aldhizer, G. R., & Juras, P. (2015). Improving the effectiveness and efficiency of health-care delivery systems. *The CPA Journal, 85*(1), 66.

Alhassan, R. K., Nketiah-Amponsah, E., & Arhinful, D. K. (2016). A review of the National Health Insurance Scheme in Ghana: What are the sustainability threats and prospects? *PLoS One, 11*(11), e0165151.

Alsan, M., Bloom, D., Canning, D., & Jamison, D. (2007). The consequences of population health for economic performance. In *Health, economic development and household poverty* (pp. 21–39). Routledge.

Alves, J., Peralta, S., & Perelman, J. (2013). Efficiency and equity consequences of decentralization in health: An economic perspective. *Revista Portuguesa de Saúde Pública, 31*(1), 74–83.

Amimo, F., Lambert, B., Magit, A., & Hashizume, M. (2021). A review of prospective pathways and impacts of COVID-19 on the accessibility, safety, quality, and affordability of essential medicines and vaccines for universal health coverage in Africa. *Globalization and Health, 17*(1), 1–15.

Arhin, K., Oteng-Abayie, E. F., & Novignon, J. (2023). Assessing the efficiency of health systems in achieving the universal health coverage goal: Evidence from Sub-Saharan Africa. *Health Economics Review, 13*(1), 1–16.

Armocida, B., Formenti, B., Palestra, F., Ussai, S., & Missoni, E. (2020). COVID-19: Universal health coverage now more than ever. *Journal of Global Health, 10*(1), PMC7211420.

Asah, F., & Nielsen, P. (2016). An integrated health management information system a missing block in achieving universal health coverage in Cameroon?

Assefa, Y., Gelaw, Y. A., Hill, P. S., Wassie Taye, B., & Van Damme, W. (2019). Community health extension program of Ethiopia, 2003–2018: Successes and challenges toward universal coverage for primary healthcare services. *Globalization and Health, 15*(1), 1–11.

Assefa, Y., Hill, P. S., Gilks, C. F., Admassu, M., Tesfaye, D., & Van Damme, W. (2020). Primary health care contributions to universal health coverage, Ethiopia. *Bulletin of the World Health Organization, 98*(12), 894.

Assefa, Y., Hill, P. S., Gilks, C. F., Damme, W. V., Pas, R. v. d., Woldeyohannes, S., & Reid, S. (2020). Global health security and universal health coverage: Understanding convergences and divergences for a synergistic response. *PloS One, 15*(12), e0244555.

Ati, N. L. P. A. P. (2018). Public health in the decentralization era towards universal coverage.

Atkinson, S., & Haran, D. (2004). Back to basics: Does decentralization improve health system performance? Evidence from Ceará in north-east Brazil. *Bulletin of the World Health Organization, 82*, 822–827.

Atun, R. (2004). What are the advantages and disadvantages of restructuring a health care system to be more focused on primary care services?

Atun, R., De Andrade, L. O. M., Almeida, G., Cotlear, D., Dmytraczenko, T., Frenz, P., . . . Muntaner, C. (2015). Health-system reform and universal health coverage in Latin America. *The Lancet, 385*(9974), 1230–1247.

Awolude, O. A., Oyerinde, S. O., & Akinyemi, J. O. (2018). Screen and triage by community extension workers to facilitate screen and treat: Task-sharing strategy to achieve universal coverage for cervical cancer screening in Nigeria. *Journal of Global Oncology, 4*, 1–10.

Balabanova, D., McKee, M., Mills, A., Walt, G., & Haines, A. (2010). What can global health institutions do to help strengthen health systems in low income countries? *Health Research Policy and Systems, 8*(1), 1–11.

Balasubramaniam, P., Rao, N., Sharma, G., Maraganty, P., Sathyanarayana, T., Lakew, D., . . . Gatellier, K. (2018). Innovations for universal health coverage: A south-south collaboration to transform health systems in Africa and India.

Baltussen, R., Jansen, M. P., Bijlmakers, L., Tromp, N., Yamin, A. E., & Norheim, O. F. (2017). Progressive realisation of universal health coverage: What are the required processes and evidence? *BMJ Global Health, 2*(3), e000342.

Bärnighausen, T., & Sauerborn, R. (2002). One hundred and eighteen years of the German health insurance system: Are there any lessons for middle-and low-income countries? *Social Science & Medicine, 54*(10), 1559–1587.

Bates, M. J., Namisango, E., Tomeny, E., Muula, A., Squire, S. B., & Niessen, L. (2019). Palliative care within universal health coverage: The Malawi Patient-and-Carer Cancer Cost Survey. *BMJ Supportive & Palliative Care.*

Bayarsaikhan, D., Tessier, L., & Ron, A. (2022). Universal health coverage and social health protection: Policy relevance to health system financing reforms. *International Social Security Review, 75*(2), 75–95.

Bekker, L.-G., Alleyne, G., Baral, S., Cepeda, J., Daskalakis, D., Dowdy, D., . . . Garnett, G. (2018). Advancing global health and strengthening the HIV response in the era of the sustainable development goals: The International AIDS Society—Lancet Commission. *The Lancet, 392*(10144), 312–358.

Bennett, S., Ozawa, S., & Rao, K. (2010). Which path to universal health coverage. *Perspectives on the world health report.*

Berhan, Y., Ali, M., Tassew, A., & Nonogaki, A. (2022). Universal health coverage policy and progress towards the attainment of universal sexual and reproductive health and rights services in Ethiopia. *Ethiopian Journal of Health Sciences, 32*(1), 181–200.

Binyaruka, P., Patouillard, E., Powell-Jackson, T., Greco, G., Maestad, O., & Borghi, J. (2015). Effect of paying for performance on utilisation, quality, and user costs of health services in Tanzania: A controlled before and after study. *PLoS One, 10*(8), e0135013.

Blaya, J. A., Fraser, H. S., & Holt, B. (2010). E-health technologies show promise in developing countries. *Health Affairs, 29*(2), 244–251.

Bloom, G. (2019). Service delivery transformation for UHC in Asia and the Pacific. *Health Systems & Reform, 5*(1), 7–17.

Boerma, T., Eozenou, P., Evans, D., Evans, T., Kieny, M.-P., & Wagstaff, A. (2014). Monitoring progress towards universal health coverage at country and global levels. *PLoS Medicine, 11*(9), e1001731.

Bors, C., Christie, A., Gervais, D., & Wright Clayton, E. (2015). Improving access to medicines in low-income countries: A review of mechanisms. *The Journal of World Intellectual Property, 18*(1–2), 1–28.

Bossert, T. J. (2013). Decentralization of health systems: Challenges and global issues of the twenty-first century. In *Decentralizing health services: A global perspective* (pp. 199–207). Springer.

Boxall, A. m. (2010). Reforming Australia's health system, again. *Medical Journal of Australia, 192*(9), 528–530.

Brennan Ramirez, L. K., Baker, E. A., & Metzler, M. (2008). Promoting health equity; a resource to help communities address social determinants of health.

Bright, T., Felix, L., Kuper, H., & Polack, S. (2017). A systematic review of strategies to increase access to health services among children in low and middle income countries. *BMC Health Services Research, 17*(1), 1–19.

Brooks, M. I., Thabrany, H., Fox, M. P., Wirtz, V. J., Feeley, F. G., & Sabin, L. L. (2017). Health facility and skilled birth deliveries among poor women with Jamkesmas health insurance in Indonesia: A mixed-methods study. *BMC Health Services Research, 17*(1), 1–12.

Bump, J. B. (2015). The long road to universal health coverage: Historical analysis of early decisions in Germany, the United Kingdom, and the United States. *Health Systems & Reform, 1*(1), 28–38.

Cameron, R., Manske, S., Brown, K. S., Jolin, M. A., Murnaghan, D., & Lovato, C. (2007). Integrating public health policy, practice, evaluation, surveillance, and research: The school health action planning and evaluation system. *American Journal of Public Health, 97*(4), 648–654.

Campbell, J., Buchan, J., Cometto, G., David, B., Dussault, G., Fogstad, H., . . . Pablos-Méndez, A. (2013). Human resources for health and universal health coverage: Fostering equity and effective coverage. *Bulletin of the World Health Organization, 91*, 853–863.

Cerda, J. S. (1990). The draft convention on the rights of the child: New rights. *Human Rights Quarterly, 12*(1), 115–119.

Chattu, V. K., Singh, B., Pattanshetty, S., & Reddy, S. (2023). Access to medicines through global health diplomacy. *Health Promotion Perspectives, 13*(1), 40.

Chaudhry, B., Wang, J., Wu, S., Maglione, M., Mojica, W., Roth, E., . . . Shekelle, P. G. (2006). Systematic review: Impact of health information technology on quality, efficiency, and costs of medical care. *Annals of Internal Medicine, 144*(10), 742–752.

Chemouni, B. (2018). The political path to universal health coverage: Power, ideas and community-based health insurance in Rwanda. *World Development, 106*, 87–98.

Chen, J., Mullins, C. D., Novak, P., & Thomas, S. B. (2016). Personalized strategies to activate and empower patients in health care and reduce health disparities. *Health Education & Behavior, 43*(1), 25–34.

Choi, B. C. (2012). The past, present, and future of public health surveillance. *Scientifica, 2012*, 875253.

Chotchoungchatchai, S., Marshall, A. I., Witthayapipopsakul, W., Panichkriangkrai, W., Patcharanarumol, W., & Tangcharoensathien, V. (2020). Primary health care and sustainable development goals. *Bulletin of the World Health Organization, 98*(11), 792.

Cipriano, P. F., Bowles, K., Dailey, M., Dykes, P., Lamb, G., & Naylor, M. (2013). The importance of health information technology in care coordination and transitional care. *Nursing Outlook, 61*(6), 475–489.

Clarke, D., Doerr, S., Hunter, M., Schmets, G., Soucat, A., & Paviza, A. (2019). The private sector and universal health coverage. *Bulletin of the World Health Organization, 97*(6), 434.

Cobos Muñoz, D., Merino Amador, P., Monzon Llamas, L., Martinez Hernandez, D., & Santos Sancho, J. M. (2017). Decentralization of health systems in low and middle income countries: A systematic review. *International Journal of Public Health, 62*, 219–229.

Coe, G., & de Beyer, J. (2014). The imperative for health promotion in universal health coverage. *Global Health: Science and Practice, 2*(1), 10–22.

Cookson, R., Mirelman, A. J., Griffin, S., Asaria, M., Dawkins, B., Norheim, O. F., . . . Culyer, A. J. (2017). Using cost-effectiveness analysis to address health equity concerns. *Value in Health*, *20*(2), 206–212.

Corbin, J. H. (2017). Health promotion, partnership and intersectoral action. *Health Promotion International*, *32*(6), 923–929.

Craven, M. (1995). *The international covenant on economic, social and cultural rights: A perspective on its development*. Clarendon Press.

Dawson, A. J., Buchan, J., Duffield, C., Homer, C. S., & Wijewardena, K. (2014). Task shifting and sharing in maternal and reproductive health in low-income countries: A narrative synthesis of current evidence. *Health Policy and Planning*, *29*(3), 396–408.

De Maeseneer, J., Li, D., Palsdottir, B., Mash, B., Aarendonk, D., Stavdal, A., . . . Ooms, G. (2020). Universal health coverage and primary health care: The 30 by 2030 campaign. *Bulletin of the World Health Organization*, *98*(11), 812.

De Vos, P., Malaise, G., De Ceukelaire, W., Perez, D., Lefèvre, P., & Van der Stuyft, P. (2009). Participation and empowerment in Primary Health Care: From Alma Ata to the era of globalization. *Social Medicine*, *4*(2), 121–127.

Debie, A., Khatri, R. B., & Assefa, Y. (2022). Successes and challenges of health systems governance towards universal health coverage and global health security: A narrative review and synthesis of the literature. *Health Research Policy and Systems*, *20*(1), 50.

Dejene, D., Yigzaw, T., Mengistu, S., Ayalew, F., Kahsaye, M., & Woldemariam, D. (2019). Exploring health workforce regulation practices and gaps in Ethiopia: A national cross-sectional study. *Global Health Research and Policy*, *4*(1), 1–12.

Dick-Sagoe, C. (2020). Decentralization for improving the provision of public services in developing countries: A critical review. *Cogent Economics & Finance*, *8*(1), 1804036.

Dimas, C. S. (2022) Health as a right in Brazil and Argentina. In *Healthcare in Latin America* (278–295),Florida Scholarship Online, Gainesville.

Donaldson, C., Baker, R., Cheater, F., Gillespie, M., McHugh, N., & Sinclair, S. (2011). Social business, health and well-being. *Social Business*, *1*(1), 17–35.

Drury, P., Roth, S., Jones, T., Stahl, M., & Medeiros, D. (2018). Guidance for investing in digital health. ADB sustainable development working paper series.

Dwicaksono, A., & Fox, A. M. (2018). Does decentralization improve health system performance and outcomes in low-and middle-income countries? A systematic review of evidence from quantitative studies. *The Milbank Quarterly*, *96*(2), 323–368.

Ehrenkranz, P., Grimsrud, A., Holmes, C. B., Preko, P., & Rabkin, M. (2021). Expanding the vision for differentiated service delivery: A call for more inclusive and truly patient-centered care for people living with HIV. *Journal of Acquired Immune Deficiency Syndromes (1999)*, *86*(2), 147.

El Ansari, W., Newbigging, K., Roth, C., & Malik, F. (2009). The role of advocacy and interpretation services in the delivery of quality healthcare to diverse minority communities in London, United Kingdom. *Health & Social Care in the Community*, *17*(6), 636–646.

Epp, J. (1986). Achieving health for all: A framework for health promotion. *Health Promotion International*, *1*(4), 419–428.

Eregata, G. T., Hailu, A., Geletu, Z. A., Memirie, S. T., Johansson, K. A., Stenberg, K., . . . Norheim, O. F. (2020). Revision of the Ethiopian essential health service package: An explication of the process and methods used. *Health Systems & Reform*, *6*(1), e1829313.

Erku, D., Khatri, R., Endalamaw, A., Wolka, E., Nigatu, F., Zewdie, A., & Assefa, Y. (2023a). Community engagement initiatives in primary health care to achieve universal health coverage: A realist synthesis of scoping review. *PloS One*, *18*(5), e0285222.

Erku, D., Khatri, R., Endalamaw, A., Wolka, E., Nigatu, F., Zewdie, A., & Assefa, Y. (2023b). Digital health interventions to improve access to and quality of primary health care services: A scoping review. *International Journal of Environmental Research and Public Health*, *20*(19), 6854.

Erondu, N. A., Martin, J., Marten, R., Ooms, G., Yates, R., & Heymann, D. L. (2018). Building the case for embedding global health security into universal health coverage: A proposal for a unified health system that includes public health. *The Lancet*, *392*(10156), 1482–1486.

Etiaba, E., Onwujekwe, O., Honda, A., Ibe, O., Uzochukwu, B., & Hanson, K. (2018). Strategic purchasing for universal health coverage: Examining the purchaser–provider relationship within a social health insurance scheme in Nigeria. *BMJ Global Health*, *3*(5), e000917.

Falkingham, J. (2004). Poverty, out-of-pocket payments and access to health care: Evidence from Tajikistan. *Social Science & Medicine*, *58*(2), 247–258.

Fan, V. Y., & Savedoff, W. D. (2014). The health financing transition: A conceptual framework and empirical evidence. *Social Science & Medicine*, *105*, 112–121.

Fantaye, A. W., & Yaya, S. (2019). Universal health coverage and facilitation of equitable access to care in Africa. *Frontiers in Public Health*, *7*, 102.

Ford, N., Ball, A., Baggaley, R., Vitoria, M., Low-Beer, D., Penazzato, M., . . . Doherty, M. (2018). The WHO public health approach to HIV treatment and care: Looking back and looking ahead. *The Lancet Infectious Diseases*, *18*(3), e76–e86.

Fox, A. M., & Reich, M. R. (2015). The politics of universal health coverage in low and middle-income countries: A framework for evaluation and action. *Journal of Health Politics, Policy and Law*, *40*(5), 1023–1060.

Franz, C., & Ghebreyesus, T. A. (2019). *The road to universal health coverage: Innovation, equity, and the new health economy.* JHU Press.

Frenk, J. (2009). Strengthening health systems to promote security. *The Lancet*, *373*(9682), 2181–2182.

Frenk, J., & De Ferranti, D. (2012). Universal health coverage: Good health, good economics. *The Lancet*, *380*(9845), 862–864.

Frenk, J., & Gómez-Dantés, O. (2018). Health systems in Latin America: The search for universal health coverage. *Archives of Medical Research*, *49*(2), 79–83.

Fusheini, A., & Eyles, J. (2016). Achieving universal health coverage in South Africa through a district health system approach: Conflicting ideologies of health care provision. *BMC Health Services Research*, *16*, 1–11.

Gilks, C. F., Crowley, S., Ekpini, R., Gove, S., Perriens, J., Souteyrand, Y., . . . De Cock, K. (2006). The WHO public-health approach to antiretroviral treatment against HIV in resource-limited settings. *The Lancet*, *368*(9534), 505–510.

Gillies, P. (1998). Effectiveness of alliances and partnerships for health promotion. *Health Promotion International*, 99–120.

Giovanella, L., Mendoza-Ruiz, A., Pilar, A. d. C. A., Rosa, M. C. d., Martins, G. B., Santos, I. S., . . . Silva, P. O. d. (2018). Universal health system and universal health coverage: Assumptions and strategies. *Ciencia & Saude Coletiva*, *23*, 1763–1776.

Glassman, A., Giedion, U., & Smith, P. C. (2017). *What's in, what's out: Designing benefits for universal health coverage.* Brookings Institution Press.

González Anaya, J. A., & García Cuéllar, R. (2015). The transformation of the Mexican Social Security Institute (IMSS): Progress and challenges. *Health Systems & Reform,* *1*(3), 189–199.

Gostin, L. O. (2021). The legal determinants of health: How can we achieve universal health coverage and what does it mean? *International Journal of Health Policy and Management,* *10*(1), 1.

Greer, S. L., & Méndez, C. A. (2015). Universal health coverage: A political struggle and governance challenge. *American Journal of Public Health,* *105*(S5), S637–S639.

Gröne, O., & Garcia-Barbero, M. (2001). Integrated care: A position paper of the WHO European office for integrated health care services. *International Journal of Integrated Care,* *1*, e21.

Gurewich, D., Garg, A., & Kressin, N. R. (2020). Addressing social determinants of health within healthcare delivery systems: A framework to ground and inform health outcomes. *Journal of General Internal Medicine,* *35*, 1571–1575.

Haakenstad, A., Irvine, C. M. S., Knight, M., Bintz, C., Aravkin, A. Y., Zheng, P., . . . Adebayo, O. M. (2022). Measuring the availability of human resources for health and its relationship to universal health coverage for 204 countries and territories from 1990 to 2019: A systematic analysis for the Global Burden of Disease Study 2019. *The Lancet,* *399*(10341), 2129–2154.

Habtemariam, M. K., & Semegn, S. T. (2018). Setting health sector priorities: A brief overview of Ethiopia's experience. *Cost Effectiveness and Resource Allocation,* *16*(1), 1–3.

Hailu, A., Eregata, G. T., Stenberg, K., & Norheim, O. F. (2021). Is universal health coverage affordable? Estimated costs and fiscal space analysis for the Ethiopian essential health services package. *Health Systems & Reform,* *7*(1), e1870061.

Haldane, V., Chuah, F. L., Srivastava, A., Singh, S. R., Koh, G. C., Seng, C. K., & Legido-Quigley, H. (2019). Community participation in health services development, implementation, and evaluation: A systematic review of empowerment, health, community, and process outcomes. *PloS One,* *14*(5), e0216112.

Han, S. M., Rahman, M. M., Rahman, M. S., Swe, K. T., Palmer, M., Sakamoto, H., . . . Shibuya, K. (2018). Progress towards universal health coverage in Myanmar: A national and subnational assessment. *The Lancet Global Health,* *6*(9), e989-e997.

Haregu, T. N., Setswe, G., Elliott, J., & Oldenburg, B. (2014). National responses to HIV/AIDS and non-communicable diseases in developing countries: Analysis of strategic parallels and differences. *Journal of Public Health Research,* *3*(1), 99.

Harries, A., Lienhardt, C., Dye, C., Evans, D., McManus, J., Terry, R., . . . Organization, W. H. (2015). Research for universal health coverage: World health report 2013.

Hashimoto, K., Adrien, L., & Rajkumar, S. (2020). Moving towards universal health coverage in Haiti. *Health Systems & Reform,* *6*(1), e1719339.

Helliwell, J. F., & Putnam, R. D. (2004). The social context of well-being. *Philosophical Transactions of the Royal Society of London. Series B: Biological Sciences,* *359*(1449), 1435–1446.

Heymann, J., & Hertzman, C. (2006). Healthier societies: An introduction. *Healthier Societies: From Analysis to Action,* 3–7.

Hill, P. S. (2018). Primary health care and universal health coverage: Competing discourses? *The Lancet,* *392*(10156), 1374–1375.

Ho, C. J., Khalid, H., Skead, K., & Wong, J. (2022). The politics of universal health coverage. *The Lancet, 399*(10340), 2066–2074.

Hogan, D. R., Stevens, G. A., Hosseinpoor, A. R., & Boerma, T. (2018). Monitoring universal health coverage within the sustainable development goals: Development and baseline data for an index of essential health services. *The Lancet Global Health, 6*(2), e152–e168.

Hort, K., Jayasuriya, R., & Dayal, P. (2017). The link between UHC reforms and health system governance: Lessons from Asia. *Journal of Health Organization and Management, 31*(3), 270–285.

Horton, R., & Das, P. (2015). Universal health coverage: Not why, what, or when—but how? *The Lancet, 385*(9974), 1156–1157.

Hussain, R., & Arif, S. (2021). Universal health coverage and COVID-19: Recent developments and implications. *Journal of Pharmaceutical Policy and Practice, 14*(1), 1–4.

Hussein, R. (2015). A review of realizing the Universal Health Coverage (UHC) goals by 2030: Part 2-what is the role of ehealth and technology? *Journal of Medical Systems, 39*, 1–10.

Ikegami, N. (2014). *Universal health coverage for inclusive and sustainable development: Lessons from Japan.* World Bank Publications.

Jabeen, R., Rabbani, U., & Abbas, N. (2021). Financing mechanisms applied for successful universal health coverage in Malaysia, Thailand and Singapore-Lessons for Pakistan.

Jaca, A., Malinga, T., Iwu-Jaja, C. J., Nnaji, C. A., Okeibunor, J. C., Kamuya, D., & Wiysonge, C. S. (2022). Strengthening the health system as a strategy to achieving a universal health coverage in underprivileged communities in Africa: A scoping review. *International Journal of Environmental Research and Public Health, 19*(1), 587.

Jackson, S. F., Perkins, F., Khandor, E., Cordwell, L., Hamann, S., & Buasai, S. (2006). Integrated health promotion strategies: A contribution to tackling current and future health challenges. *Health Promotion International, 21*(suppl_1), 75–83.

Jain, V., & Alam, A. (2017). Redefining universal health coverage in the age of global health security. *BMJ Global Health, 2*(2), e000255.

Joarder, T., Chaudhury, T. Z., & Mannan, I. (2019). Universal health coverage in Bangladesh: Activities, challenges, and suggestions. *Advances in Public Health.*

Karamagi, H. C., Tumusiime, P., Titi-Ofei, R., Droti, B., Kipruto, H., Nabyonga-Orem, J., . . . Cabore, J. W. (2021). Towards universal health coverage in the WHO African Region: Assessing health system functionality, incorporating lessons from COVID-19. *BMJ Global Health, 6*(3), e004618.

Kelsall, T., Hart, T., & Laws, E. (2016). Political settlements and pathways to universal health coverage. *London: Overseas Development Institute*, 1–32.

Khatri, R., Endalamaw, A., Erku, D., Wolka, E., Nigatu, F., Zewdie, A., & Assefa, Y. (2023). Continuity and care coordination of primary health care: A scoping review. *BMC Health Services Research, 23*(1), 750.

Khatri, R. B., Erku, D., Endalamaw, A., Wolka, E., Nigatu, F., Zewdie, A., & Assefa, Y. (2023). Multisectoral actions in primary health care: A realist synthesis of scoping review. *PloS One, 18*(8), e0289816.

Kieny, M. P., Bekedam, H., Dovlo, D., Fitzgerald, J., Habicht, J., Harrison, G., . . . Mirza, Z. (2017). Strengthening health systems for universal health coverage and sustainable development. *Bulletin of the World Health Organization, 95*(7), 537.

Kieny, M. P., & Evans, D. B. (2013). Universal health coverage. *EMHJ-Eastern Mediterranean Health Journal, 19*(4), 305–306, 2013.

King, M. (1966). Medical care in developing countries. A primer on the medicine of poverty and a symposium from Makerere.

Kirigia, J. M., Kathyola, D. D., Muula, A. S., & Ota, M. M. O. (2015). National health research system in Malawi: Dead, moribund, tepid or flourishing? *Bmc Health Services Research, 15*, 1–14.

Knaul, F., Bhadelia, A., Atun, R., De Lima, L., & Radbruch, L. (2019). Palliative care: An essential facet of universal health coverage. *The Lancet Global Health, 7*(11), e1488.

Knaul, F. M., Bhadelia, A., Atun, R., & Frenk, J. (2015). Achieving effective universal health coverage and diagonal approaches to care for chronic illnesses. *Health Affairs, 34*(9), 1514–1522.

Kraef, C., & Kallestrup, P. (2019). After the Astana declaration: Is comprehensive primary health care set for success this time? *BMJ Global Health, 4*(6), 1871.

Kruk, M. E., Myers, M., Varpilah, S. T., & Dahn, B. T. (2015). What is a resilient health system? Lessons from Ebola. *The Lancet, 385*(9980), 1910–1912.

Kushitor, M. K., Biney, A. A., Wright, K., Phillips, J. F., Awoonor-Williams, J. K., & Bawah, A. A. (2019). A qualitative appraisal of stakeholders' perspectives of a community-based primary health care program in rural Ghana. *BMC Health Services Research, 19*(1), 1–13.

Kutzin, J. (2008). Health financing policy: A guide for decision-makers. *Health financing policy paper*. Copenhagen, WHO Regional Office for Europe, 24.

Kutzin, J. (2013). Health financing for universal coverage and health system performance: Concepts and implications for policy. *Bulletin of the World Health Organization, 91*, 602–611.

Kutzin, J., & Sparkes, S. P. (2016). Health systems strengthening, universal health coverage, health security and resilience. *Bulletin of the World Health Organization, 94*(1), 2.

Lagomarsino, G., Garabrant, A., Adyas, A., Muga, R., & Otoo, N. (2012). Moving towards universal health coverage: Health insurance reforms in nine developing countries in Africa and Asia. *The Lancet, 380*(9845), 933–943.

Lal, A., Abdalla, S. M., Chattu, V. K., Erondu, N. A., Lee, T.-L., Singh, S., . . . Phelan, A. (2022). Pandemic preparedness and response: Exploring the role of universal health coverage within the global health security architecture. *The Lancet Global Health, 10*(11), e1675–e1683.

Lal, A., Erondu, N. A., Heymann, D. L., Gitahi, G., & Yates, R. (2021). Fragmented health systems in COVID-19: Rectifying the misalignment between global health security and universal health coverage. *The Lancet, 397*(10268), 61–67.

Lantz, J. M., Fullerton, J. T., Harshburger, R. J., & Sadler, G. R. (2001). Promoting screening and early detection of cancer in men. *Nursing & Health Sciences, 3*(4), 189–196.

Lê, G., Morgan, R., Bestall, J., Featherstone, I., Veale, T., & Ensor, T. (2016). Can service integration work for universal health coverage? Evidence from around the globe. *Health Policy, 120*(4), 406–419.

Letebo, M., & Shiferaw, F. (2016). Adapting HIV patient and program monitoring tools for chronic non-communicable diseases in Ethiopia. *Globalization and Health, 12*(1), 26.

Lewis, M., & Pettersson Gelander, G. (2009). Governance in health care delivery: Raising performance. *World Bank Policy Research Working Paper* (5074).

Liaropoulos, L., & Goranitis, I. (2015). Health care financing and the sustainability of health systems. *International Journal for Equity in Health, 14*(1), 1–4.

Lim, M. Y., Kamaruzaman, H. F., Wu, O., & Geue, C. (2023). Health financing challenges in Southeast Asian countries for universal health coverage: A systematic review. *Archives of Public Health, 81*(1), 1–12.

Lygidakis, C., McLoughlin, C., & Patel, K. (2016). *Achieving universal health coverage: Technology for innovative primary health care education.*

Macdonald, V., Verster, A., Seale, A., Baggaley, R., & Ball, A. (2019). Universal health coverage and key populations. *Current Opinion in HIV and AIDS, 14*(5), 433–438.

Maeda, A., Araujo, E., Cashin, C., Harris, J., Ikegami, N., & Reich, M. R. (2014). *Universal health coverage for inclusive and sustainable development: A synthesis of 11 country case studies.* World Bank Publications.

Mao, W., Tang, Y., Tran, T., Pender, M., Khanh, P. N., & Tang, S. (2020). Advancing universal health coverage in China and Vietnam: Lessons for other countries. *BMC Public Health, 20*(1), 1–9.

Marmot, M., Friel, S., Bell, R., Houweling, T. A., Taylor, S., & Health, C. o. S. D. o. (2008). Closing the gap in a generation: Health equity through action on the social determinants of health. *The Lancet, 372*(9650), 1661–1669.

Mathauer, I., Torres, L. V., Kutzin, J., Jakab, M., & Hanson, K. (2020). Pooling financial resources for universal health coverage: Options for reform. *Bulletin of the World Health Organization, 98*(2), 132.

Mazaba, M., Mwaba, P., Droti, B., Kagulura, S., Makasa, C., Masaninga, F., . . . Mufunda, J. (2016). Leveraging existing laboratory capacity towards universal health coverage: A case of Zambian laboratory services. *Medical Journal of Zambia, 43*(2), 88–93.

Mboi, N. (2015). Indonesia: On the way to universal health care. *Health Systems & Reform, 1*(2), 91–97.

McIntyre, D., Obse, A. G., Barasa, E. W., & Ataguba, J. E. (2018). Challenges in financing universal health coverage in sub-Saharan Africa. In *Oxford research encyclopedia of economics and finance.*

Meleis, A. I. (1992). Community participation and involvement: Theoretical and empirical issues. *Health Services Management Research, 5*(1), 5–16.

Mendes, L. d. S., & Almeida, P. F. d. (2020). Do primary and specialized care physicians know and use coordination mechanisms? *Rev Saude Publica, 54*, 121.

Misganaw, A. (2020). Implications of forecasted disease burden on envisioning health strategies in Ethiopia; Findings from Global Burden of Disease 2017 Forecasting Study.

Moreno-Serra, R., & Smith, P. C. (2012). Does progress towards universal health coverage improve population health? *The Lancet, 380*(9845), 917–923.

Morgan, L. M. (2001). Community participation in health: Perpetual allure, persistent challenge. *Health Policy and Planning, 16*(3), 221–230.

Morgan, R., Ensor, T., & Waters, H. (2016). Performance of private sector health care: Implications for universal health coverage. *The Lancet, 388*(10044), 606–612.

Mpofu, M., Semo, B.-w., Grignon, J., Lebelonyane, R., Ludick, S., Matshediso, E., . . . Ledikwe, J. H. (2014). Strengthening monitoring and evaluation (M&E) and building sustainable health information systems in resource limited countries: Lessons learned from an M&E task-shifting initiative in Botswana. *BMC Public Health, 14*, 1–8.

Mullan, Z. (2016). Transforming health care in Ethiopia. *The Lancet Global Health, 4*(1), e1.

Muzaka, V. (2017). Lessons from Brazil: On the difficulties of building a universal health care system. *Journal of Global Health, 7*(1), 010303.

Myint, C.-Y., Pavlova, M., Thein, K.-N.-N., & Groot, W. (2019). A systematic review of the health-financing mechanisms in the Association of Southeast Asian Nations countries and the People's Republic of China: Lessons for the move towards universal health coverage. *PloS One, 14*(6), e0217278.

Nde, C. J., Raymond, A., & Saidou, Y. (2019). Progress towards universal health coverage: Is Cameroon investing enough in primary care. *Universal J Public Health, 7*(4), 171–178.

Neelsen, S., & O'Donnell, O. (2017). Progressive universalism? The impact of targeted coverage on health care access and expenditures in Peru. *Health Economics, 26*(12), e179–e203.

Niessen, L. W., & Squire, S. B. (2019). Universal health coverage and chronic conditions. *The Lancet Global Health, 7*(10), e1290–e1292.

Norheim, O. F. (2015). Ethical perspective: Five unacceptable trade-offs on the path to universal health coverage. *International Journal of Health Policy and Management, 4*(11), 711.

Novignon, J., Lanko, C., & Arthur, E. (2021). Political economy and the pursuit of universal health coverage in Ghana: A case study of the National Health Insurance Scheme. *Health Policy and Planning, 36*(Supplement_1), i14–i21.

Nyandekwe, M., Nzayirambaho, M., & Kakoma, J. B. (2014). Universal health coverage in Rwanda: Dream or reality. *The Pan African Medical Journal, 17*, 232.

Odoch, W. D., Senkubuge, F., & Hongoro, C. (2021). How has sustainable development goals declaration influenced health financing reforms for universal health coverage at the country level? A scoping review of literature. *Globalization and Health, 17*(1), 1–13.

Okech, T. C. (2017). Devolution of public health care services in Kenya and its implication on universal health coverage. *IOSR Journal of Pharmacy, 7*(5/1), 9–23.

Okpani, A. I., & Abimbola, S. (2015). Operationalizing universal health coverage in Nigeria through social health insurance. *Nigerian Medical Journal: Journal of the Nigeria Medical Association, 56*(5), 305.

Oni, T., Mogo, E., Ahmed, A., & Davies, J. I. (2019). Breaking down the silos of Universal Health Coverage: Towards systems for the primary prevention of non-communicable diseases in Africa. *BMJ Global Health, 4*(4), e001717.

Onoka, C. A., Hanson, K., & Hanefeld, J. (2015). Towards universal coverage: A policy analysis of the development of the National Health Insurance Scheme in Nigeria. *Health Policy and Planning, 30*(9), 1105–1117.

Ooms, G., Beiersmann, C., Flores, W., Hanefeld, J., Müller, O., Mulumba, M., . . . Jahn, A. (2017). Synergies and tensions between universal health coverage and global health security: Why we need a second 'Maximizing Positive Synergies' initiative. *BMJ Global Health, 2*(1), e000217. https://doi.org/10.1136/bmjgh-2016-000217

Ooms, G., Ottersen, T., Jahn, A., & Agyepong, I. A. (2018). Addressing the fragmentation of global health: The Lancet Commission on synergies between universal health coverage, health security, and health promotion. *The Lancet, 392*(10153), 1098–1099.

Pablos-Mendez, A., Cavanaugh, K., & Ly, C. (2016). The new era of health goals: Universal health coverage as a pathway to the sustainable development goals. *Health Systems & Reform, 2*(1), 15–17.

Pai, M., & Kohli, M. (2019). Essential diagnostics: A key element of universal health coverage. *Dr. Sulaiman Al Habib Medical Journal*, *1*(00), 3–7.

Paolucci, F., Redekop, K., Fouda, A., & Fiorentini, G. (2017). Decision making and priority setting: The evolving path towards universal health coverage. *Applied Health Economics and Health Policy*, *15*, 697–706.

Piot, P., Karim, S. S. A., Hecht, R., Legido-Quigley, H., Buse, K., Stover, J., . . . Dybul, M. (2015). Defeating AIDS—advancing global health. *The Lancet*, *386*(9989), 171–218.

Pisani, E., Olivier Kok, M., & Nugroho, K. (2017). Indonesia's road to universal health coverage: A political journey. *Health Policy and Planning*, *32*(2), 267–276.

Pratiwi, A. B., Setiyaningsih, H., Kok, M. O., Hoekstra, T., Mukti, A. G., & Pisani, E. (2021). Is Indonesia achieving universal health coverage? Secondary analysis of national data on insurance coverage, health spending and service availability. *BMJ Open*, *11*(10), e050565.

Preker, A. S., Cotlear, D., Kwon, S., Atun, R., & Avila, C. (2021). Universal health care in middle-income countries: Lessons from four countries. *Journal of Global Health*, *11*, 16004.

Ranabhat, C. L., Jakovljevic, M. M., & Kim, C.-B. (2021). COVID-19 Pandemic: An opportunity for universal health coverage? *Frontiers in Public Health*, *9*, 1057.

Rannan-Eliya, R. P., Anuranga, C., Manual, A., Sararaks, S., Jailani, A. S., Hamid, A. J., . . . Darzi, A. (2016). Improving health care coverage, equity, and financial protection through a hybrid system: Malaysia's experience. *Health Affairs*, *35*(5), 838–846.

Rao, K. D., Makimoto, S., Peters, M., Leung, G. M., Bloom, G., & Katsuma, Y. (2019). Vulnerable populations and universal health coverage. *Leave no one behind: Time for specifics on the sustainable development goals*.

Rao, K. D., Paina, L., Ingabire, M.-G., & Shroff, Z. C. (2018). Contracting non-state providers for universal health coverage: Learnings from Africa, Asia, and Eastern Europe. *International Journal for Equity in Health*, *17*(1), 1–9.

Rashidian, A. (1995). Effective health information systems for delivering the Sustainable Development Goals and the universal health coverage agenda. *Information for Authors*, *1*.

Remington, P. L., & Nelson, D. E. (2010). Communicating public health surveillance information for action. *Principles and practice of public health surveillance*, 3rd edn (pp. 146–165). Oxford University Press, Oxford.

Reta, A., & Simachew, A. (2018). The role of private health sector for tuberculosis control in Debre Markos town, Northwest Ethiopia. *Advances in Medicine*, *2018*, 8697470.

Rifkin, S. B. (2003). A framework linking community empowerment and health equity: It is a matter of CHOICE. *Journal of Health, Population and Nutrition*, *21*(3), 168–180.

Rifkin, S. B. (2009). Lessons from community participation in health programmes: A review of the post Alma-Ata experience. *International Health*, *1*(1), 31–36.

Rifkin, S. B. (2018). Health for all and primary health care, 1978–2018: A historical perspective on policies and programs over 40 years. In *Oxford research encyclopedia of global public health*.

Robert, E., Zongo, S., Rajan, D., & Ridde, V. (2022). Contributing to collaborative health governance in Africa: A realist evaluation of the universal health coverage partnership. *BMC Health Services Research*, *22*(1), 1–19.

Rozenblum, R., Miller, P., Pearson, D., Marielli, A., Grando, M., & Bates, D. (2015). Patient-centered healthcare, patient engagement and health information technology:

The perfect storm. In *Information technology for patient empowerment in healthcare* (pp. 3–22).Walter de Gruyter Inc, Berlin.

Rusakaniko, S., Makanga, M., Ota, M. O., Bockarie, M., Banda, G., Okeibunor, J., . . . Kirigia, J. M. (2019). Strengthening national health research systems in the WHO African Region–progress towards universal health coverage. *Globalization and Health*, *15*, 1–14.

Rushton, S. (2011). Global health security: Security for whom? Security from what? *Political Studies*, *59*(4), 779–796.

Russell, E., Johnson, B., Larsen, H., Novilla, M. L. B., Olmen, J. v., & Swanson, R. C. (2013). Health systems in context: A systematic review of the integration of the social determinants of health within health systems frameworks. *Revista Panamericana de Salud Publica*, *34*(6), 461–467.

Sacks, E., Schleiff, M., Were, M., Chowdhury, A. M., & Perry, H. B. (2020). Communities, universal health coverage and primary health care. *Bulletin of the World Health Organization*, *98*(11), 773.

Sahay, S., Nielsen, P., & Aanestad, M. (2018). Institutionalizing information systems for universal health coverage in primary health care and the need for new forms of institutional work. *Communications of the Association for Information Systems*.

Samuel, M., Irene, M., & Kenny, K. (2020). Readiness of primary health care diagnostic laboratory services to support UHC programme in Kenya: A case study of three counties. *Journal of Health and Environmental Research*, *6*(4), 128–142.

Sarker, M., Hossain, P., Ahmed, S. T., Barua, M., Sutradhar, I., & Ahmed, S. M. (2022). A critical look at synergies and fragmentations of universal health coverage, global health security, and health promotion in delivery of frontline health care services: A case study of Bangladesh. *The Lancet Regional Health-Southeast Asia*, *7*, 100087.

Savedoff, W. D., de Ferranti, D., Smith, A. L., & Fan, V. (2012). Political and economic aspects of the transition to universal health coverage. *The Lancet*, *380*(9845), 924–932.

Savedoff, W. D., & Smith, A. L. (2011). *Achieving universal health coverage: Learning from Chile, Japan, Malaysia and Sweden*. Results for Development Institute, Washington, DC.

Savel, T. G., Foldy, S., Control, C. f. D., & Prevention. (2012). The role of public health informatics in enhancing public health surveillance. *MMWR Surveillance Summaries*, *61*(2), 20–24.

Sayinzoga, F., Tetui, M., van der Velden, K., van Dillen, J., & Bijlmakers, L. (2019). Understanding variation in health service coverage and maternal health outcomes among districts in Rwanda–A qualitative study of local health workers' perceptions. *PLoS One*, *14*(10), e0223357.

Shi, L., Tsai, J., & Kao, S. (2009). Public health, social determinants of health, and public policy. *The Journal of Medical Sciences*, *29*(2), 43–59.

Shiferaw, F., Letebo, M., Misganaw, A., Feleke, Y., Gelibo, T., Getachew, T., Defar, A., Assefa, A., Bekele, A., & Amenu, K. (2018). Non-communicable diseases in Ethiopia: Disease burden, gaps in health care delivery and strategic directions. *Ethiopian Journal of Health Development*, *32*(3).

Shilton, T., & Barry, M. M. (2022). The critical role of health promotion for effective universal health coverage. *Glob Health Promotion*, *29*(1), 92–95.

Siddiqi, S., Masud, T. I., Nishtar, S., Peters, D. H., Sabri, B., Bile, K. M., & Jama, M. A. (2009). Framework for assessing governance of the health system in developing countries: Gateway to good governance. *Health Policy*, *90*(1), 13–25.

Sobel, H. L., Huntington, D., & Temmerman, M. (2016). Quality at the centre of universal health coverage. *Health Policy and Planning, 31*(4), 547–549.

Starfield, B., Shi, L., & Macinko, J. (2005). Contribution of primary care to health systems and health. *The Milbank Quarterly, 83*(3), 457–502.

Tadesse, A. W., Gurmu, K. K., Kebede, S. T., & Habtemariam, M. K. (2021). Analyzing efforts to synergize the global health agenda of universal health coverage, health security and health promotion: A case-study from Ethiopia. *Globalization and Health, 17*(1), 1–13.

Takahashi, Y. (2016). Primary health care and universal health coverage in certain international instruments and the implementation-The case of Japan. *Asian Journal of WTO & International Health Law and Policy, 11*, 477.

Takaku, R., Bessho, S., Nishimura, S., & Ikegami, N. (2014). Fiscal disparities among social health insurance programs in Japan. *Universal health coverage for inclusive and sustainable development: Lessons from Japan* (pp. 41–55). World Bank, Washington, DC.

Tan, K. B., & Earn Lee, C. (2019). Integration of primary care with hospital services for sustainable universal health coverage in Singapore. *Health Systems & Reform, 5*(1), 18–23.

Tan, S. Y., Wu, X., & Yang, W. (2019). Impacts of the type of social health insurance on health service utilisation and expenditures: Implications for a unified system in China. *Health Economics, Policy and Law, 14*(4), 468–486.

Tanahashi, T. (1978). Health service coverage and its evaluation. *Bulletin of the World Health Organization, 56*(2), 295.

Tandon, A., & Reddy, K. S. (2021). Redistribution and the health financing transition. *Journal of Global Health, 11*, 16002.

Tangcharoensathien, V., Limwattananon, S., Patcharanarumol, W., Thammatacharee, J., Jongudomsuk, P., & Sirilak, S. (2015). Achieving universal health coverage goals in Thailand: The vital role of strategic purchasing. *Health Policy and Planning, 30*(9), 1152–1161.

Tangcharoensathien, V., Patcharanarumol, W., Kulthanmanusorn, A., & Pablos-Mendez, A. (2021). Paths towards universal health coverage: Beyond political commitments. *Journal of Global Health, 11*, 16002.

Tangcharoensathien, V., Patcharanarumol, W., Panichkriangkrai, W., & Sommanustweechai, A. (2017). Policy choices for progressive realization of universal health coverage: Comment on "Ethical perspective: Five unacceptable trade-offs on the path to universal health coverage". *International Journal of Health Policy and Management, 6*(2), 107.

Tangcharoensathien, V., Pitayarangsarit, S., Patcharanarumol, W., Prakongsai, P., Sumalee, H., Tosanguan, J., & Mills, A. (2013). Promoting universal financial protection: How the Thai universal coverage scheme was designed to ensure equity. *Health Research Policy and Systems, 11*(1), 1–9.

Tangcharoensathien, V., Thammatach-Aree, J., Witthayapipopsakul, W., Viriyathorn, S., Kulthanmanusorn, A., & Patcharanarumol, W. (2020). Political economy of Thailand's tax-financed universal coverage scheme. *Bulletin of the World Health Organization, 98*(2), 140.

Tangcharoensathien, V., Tisayaticom, K., Suphanchaimat, R., Vongmongkol, V., Viriyathorn, S., & Limwattananon, S. (2020). Financial risk protection of Thailand's universal health coverage: Results from series of national household surveys between 1996 and 2015. *International Journal for Equity in Health, 19*, 1–12.

Tangcharoensathien, V., Witthayapipopsakul, W., Panichkriangkrai, W., Patcharanaru-mol, W., & Mills, A. (2018). Health systems development in Thailand: A solid platform for successful implementation of universal health coverage. *The Lancet, 391*(10126), 1205–1223.

Thakur, R., Hsu, S. H., & Fontenot, G. (2012). Innovation in healthcare: Issues and future trends. *Journal of Business Research, 65*(4), 562–569.

The Word Bank. (1993). *World development report 1993: Investing in health.* World Bank, New York.

Thomson, S., Foubister, T., Figueras, J., Kutzin, J., Permanand, G., Bryndová, L., & Organization, W. H. (2009). Addressing financial sustainability in health systems.

Thornton, R. L., Glover, C. M., Cené, C. W., Glik, D. C., Henderson, J. A., & Williams, D. R. (2016). Evaluating strategies for reducing health disparities by addressing the social determinants of health. *Health Affairs, 35*(8), 1416–1423.

Tolla, M. T., Norheim, O. F., Verguet, S., Bekele, A., Amenu, K., Abdisa, S. G., & Johans-son, K. A. (2017). Out-of-pocket expenditures for prevention and treatment of cardio-vascular disease in general and specialised cardiac hospitals in Addis Ababa, Ethiopia: A cross-sectional cohort study. *BMJ Global Health, 2*(2), e000280.

Tollman, S. M., Kahn, K., Sartorius, B., Collinson, M. A., Clark, S. J., & Garenne, M. L. (2008). Implications of mortality transition for primary health care in rural South Africa: A population-based surveillance study. *The Lancet, 372*(9642), 893–901.

Tomlinson, M., Rotheram-Borus, M. J., Swartz, L., & Tsai, A. C. (2013). Scaling up mHealth: Where is the evidence? *PLoS Medicine, 10*(2), e1001382.

Tossy, T. (2014). Major challenges and constraint of integrating health information sys-tems in african countries: A Namibian experience. *International Journal of Informa-tion and Communication Technology, 4*(7), 273–279.

Tran Ngoc, C., Bigirimana, N., Muneene, D., Bataringaya, J. E., Barango, P., Eskandar, H., . . . Olu, O. (2018). Conclusions of the digital health hub of the Transform Africa Summit (2018): Strong government leadership and public-private-partnerships are key prerequisites for sustainable scale up of digital health in Africa. *BMC Proceedings, 12*(Suppl 11), 17

Tumusiime, P., Kwamie, A., Akogun, O. B., Elongo, T., & Nabyonga-Orem, J. (2019). Towards universal health coverage: Reforming the neglected district health system in Africa. *BMJ Global Health, 4*(Suppl 9), e001498.

Umeh, C. A. (2018). Challenges toward achieving universal health coverage in Ghana, Kenya, Nigeria, and Tanzania. *The International Journal of Health Planning and Man-agement, 33*(4), 794–805.

United Nations General Assembly. (1948). Universal declaration of human rights. *UN General Assembly, 302*(2), 14–25. http://www.multiculturalaustralia.edu.au/doc/unh-rights_1.pdf

United Nations General Assembly. (2012). Resolution adopted by the General Assembly on 27 July 2012.

United Nations General Assembly. (2015). Transforming our world: The 2030 Agenda for Sustainable Development. *UN Doc. A/RES/70/1 (September 25, 2015).*

Uzochukwu, B., Onwujekwe, E., Mbachu, C., Okeke, C., Molyneux, S., & Gilson, L. (2018). Accountability mechanisms for implementing a health financing option: The case of the basic health care provision fund (BHCPF) in Nigeria. *International Journal for Equity in Health, 17*, 1–16.

Van Doorslaer, E., O'Donnell, O., Rannan-Eliya, R. P., Somanathan, A., Adhikari, S. R., Akkazieva, B., . . . Huq, M. N. (2005). Paying out-of-pocket for health care in Asia: Catastrophic and poverty impact. *Erasmus University, Rotterdam and IPS, Colombo.*

Verguet, S., Hailu, A., Eregata, G. T., Memirie, S. T., Johansson, K. A., & Norheim, O. F. (2021). Toward universal health coverage in the post-COVID-19 era. *Nature Medicine, 27*(3), 380–387.

Verrecchia, R., Thompson, R., & Yates, R. (2019). Universal health coverage and public health: A truly sustainable approach. *The Lancet Public Health, 4*(1), e10–e11.

Wang, H., Juma, M. A., Rosemberg, N., & Ulisubisya, M. M. (2018a). Progressive Pathway to Universal Health Coverage in Tanzania.

Wang, H., Juma, M. A., Rosemberg, N., & Ulisubisya, M. M. (2018b). Progressive pathway to universal health coverage in Tanzania: A call for preferential resource allocation targeting the poor. *Health Systems & Reform, 4*(4), 279–283.

Watkins, D. A., Jamison, D. T., Mills, T., Atun, T., Danforth, K., Glassman, A., . . . Norheim, O. F. (2018). Universal health coverage and essential packages of care. In Disease control priorities: Improving health and reducing poverty, 3rd edn. World Bank, Washington, DC.

Webster, C. (2002). *The national health service: A political history.* Oxford University Press, Oxford.

White, F. (2015). Primary health care and public health: Foundations of universal health systems. *Medical Principles and Practice, 24*(2), 103–116.

Whiting, S., Dalipanda, T., Postma, S., de Lorenzo, A. J., & Aumua, A. (2016). Moving towards universal health coverage through the development of integrated service delivery packages for primary health care in the Solomon Islands. *International Journal of Integrated Care, 16*(1), 3.

WHO, U. (1978). Declaration of Alma-Ata: International conference on primary health care. *Alma-Ata, USSR,* 6–12.

Woolf, S. H. (2009). A closer look at the economic argument for disease prevention. *JAMA, 301*(5), 536–538.

Woolf, S. H., Jonas, S., & Kaplan-Liss, E. (2008). *Health promotion and disease prevention in clinical practice.* Lippincott Williams & Wilkins.

World Health Organisation (WHO). (2011). *Sixty-fourth world health assembly.* https://apps.who.int/gb/ebwha/pdf_files/WHA64-REC1/A64_REC1-en.pdf

World Health Organisation (WHO). (2013). Follow-up of the report of the Consultative Expert Working Group on Research and Development: Financing and coordination.

World Health Organization (WHO). (1946). The constitution of the World Health Organization.

World Health Organization (WHO). (1978a). Declaration of Alma-Ata: International Conference on Primary Health Care, Alma-Ata, USSR, 6–12 September 1978.

World Health Organization (WHO). (1978b). Declaration of Alma Ata: Report of the international conference on primary health care. *Alma Atta, USSR.*

World Health Organization (WHO). (1979). Formulating strategies for health for all by the year 2000.

World Health Organization (WHO). (1986). Ottawa charter for health promotion, 1986.

World Health Organization (WHO). (2000). The world health report 2000. Health systems: Improving performance. *Bulletin of the World Health Organization, 78*(8), 1064.

World Health Organization (WHO). (2005a). *Preventing chronic diseases: A vital investment.* World Health Organization, Geneva.

World Health Organization (WHO). (2005b). Sustainable health financing, universal coverage and social health insurance. *World Health Assembly Resolution, 58*, 139–140.

World Health Organization (WHO). (2008). The challenges of a changing world. the world health report 2008—primary health care (now more than ever).

World Health Organization (WHO). (2010). *The world health report: Health systems financing: The path to universal coverage: Executive summary.*

World Health Organization (WHO). (2015). *Health in 2015: From MDGs, millennium development goals to SDGs, sustainable development goals.* World Health Organization, Geneva.

World Health Organization (WHO). (2017a). Leave no one behind: Strengthening health systems for UHC and the SDGs in Africa.

World Health Organization (WHO). (2017b). SDGs and progress towards universal health coverage.

World Health Organization (WHO). (2018a). Essential public health functions, health systems and health security: Developing conceptual clarity and a WHO roadmap for action.

World Health Organization (WHO). (2018b). Health in All Policies as part of the primary health care agenda on multisectoral action.

World Health Organization (WHO). (2018c). Moving ahead with Universal Health Coverage and other health SDG targets in countries of the African Region.

World Health Organization (WHO). (2018d). Primary health care: Closing the gap between public health and primary care through integration.

World Health Organization (WHO). (2018e). Thirteenth general programme of work 2019–2023. *The seventy-first world health assembly.* World Health Organization, Geneva. https://www.who.int/docs/default-source/documents/gpw/who-results-framework-draft-25october2019.pdf?sfvrsn=fcee6eb2_2

World Health Organization (WHO). (2018f). A vision for primary health care in the 21st century: Towards universal health coverage and the sustainable development goals.

World Health Organization (WHO). (2021a). Building health systems resilience for universal health coverage and health security during the COVID-19 pandemic and beyond: WHO position paper.

World Health Organization (WHO). (2021b). Global strategy on digital health 2020–2025.

World Health Organization (WHO). (2021c). Principles of health benefit packages.

World Health Organization (WHO). (2023). Tracking Universal Health Coverage: 2023 Global Monitoring Report.

Yates, R. (2009). Universal health care and the removal of user fees. *The Lancet, 373*(9680), 2078–2081.

Yeoh, E.-K., Johnston, C., Chau, P. Y. K., Kiang, N., Tin, P., & Tang, J. (2019). Governance functions to accelerate progress toward universal health coverage (UHC) in the Asia-Pacific Region. *Health Systems & Reform, 5*(1), 48–58.

Yu, H. (2015). Universal health insurance coverage for 1.3 billion people: What accounts for China's success? *Health Policy, 119*(9), 1145–1152.

Zakumumpa, H., Bennett, S., & Ssengooba, F. (2019). Leveraging the lessons learned from financing HIV programs to advance the universal health coverage (UHC) agenda in the East African Community. *Global Health Research and Policy, 4*, 1–10.

Index

Note: **Bold** page numbers refer to tables and *italic* page numbers refer to figures.

For Product Safety Concerns and Information please contact our EU
representative GPSR@taylorandfrancis.com
Taylor & Francis Verlag GmbH, Kaufingerstraße 24, 80331 München, Germany